THE LINE

WHERE MEDICINE AND SPORT COLLIDE

Further Praise for Dr Richard Freeman

'I have always found Richard to be incredibly kind hearted, caring and deeply compassionate' – Mark Cavendish, Road World Champion and Tour de France multi-stage sprint champion

'Doctor Freeman is a pioneer in medical performance services in recovery and preparation for world class sports teams and athletes. In my opinion number one in his field . . .' – Mark Taylor, Performance Director

'Dr Rich's calm, professional and rational attitude gives everyone around him the confidence that all has been done for the athlete in order to be 100% able to focus on the job' – Heiko Salzwedel, Olympic men's team pursuit coach

'Not only is he a brilliant doctor who I loved working with, he was also just a great person to talk to, always understanding the human side of what can sometimes be a fickle sport' – Richie Porte, ProTour cyclist

DR RICHARD FREEMAN

THE
LINE

WHERE MEDICINE AND
SPORT COLLIDE

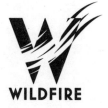

WILDFIRE

First published in 2018
by WILDFIRE
an imprint of HEADLINE PUBLISHING GROUP

1

Cataloguing in Publication Data is available from the British Library

Hardback ISBN 978 1 4722 5973 8
Trade Paperback ISBN 978 1 4722 5974 5

Typeset in Adobe Garamond Pro by Palimpsest Book Production Ltd,
Falkirk, Stirlingshire

Printed and bound in Great Britain by
Clays Ltd, Elcograf S.p.A.

Papers used by Headline are from well-managed
forests and other responsible sources.

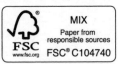

HEADLINE PUBLISHING GROUP
An Hachette UK Company
Carmelite House
50 Victoria Embankment
London EC4Y 0DZ

www.headline.co.uk
www.hachette.co.uk

For my patients in general practice and elite sport.
It's been a privilege being your doctor.

foreword

I can't promise that you'll be a better sportsperson as a result of reading this book. However, knowing Dr Richard Freeman as I do, I can promise you this: you'll be a much better prepared and informed sportsperson as a result of reading this book. And you can't say fairer than that.

He and I met a while back when I took him on as club doctor at Bolton Wanderers, and we hit it off at once. Put it this way, if there's such a thing as a chance meeting, and such a thing as a meeting of minds, our connection was what you might call a chance meeting of minds.

Like everybody else I called him Doc, same as I would with any other club medic. But where this 'Doc' differed from his predecessors was his background in what was then an emerging discipline – sports and exercise medicine – which meant that he came armed with a readiness to explore new ways of thinking that, while commonplace now, were new to football at the time. He and my trusted physiotherapist, Mark Taylor, who also had a degree in sports science, formed a great partnership.

The application of science, both in sports and in coaching, was very much my own area of interest. Whether it was on the field, preparing for the match, or refueling and recovering afterwards, I was always looking for new ways of finding the edge over the competition, always interrogating every aspect of what we were doing and asking, *Could we do that better?*

So as you can imagine, I needed someone to share my vision. And in Doc I found that someone. He didn't roll his eyes whenever I suggested something new; he came up with plenty of ideas of his own and he was a great club doctor to boot. From the everyday muscle strains and torn ligaments suffered by your average Premiership footballer, to his superlative handling of Khalilou Fadiga (about whom you can read in this book), Doc was never less than supremely competent and professional, a credit to medicine and to Bolton. Premiership football can appear to be a glamorous environment. It's easy to get your head turned, but he was never like that. To him, they were always patients before they were star players.

So I was not at all surprised that he went on to achieve such great success with British Cycling and Team Sky. However it's unfortunate that he has never received full credit for his part in the cycling team's success.

I hope that his book will see that minor injustice addressed. More importantly, I'm happy that he's chosen to share some of his wisdom and skills within these pages, so that everyone, not just elite athletes, can benefit from what is a truly unique and original approach to the business of medicine and sport.

Sam Allardyce, May 2018

Prologue

July 8 2011, the seventh stage of the Tour de France

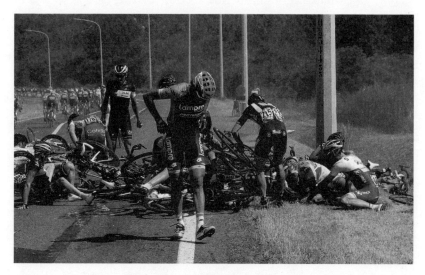

Crash, stage 3, 2015 Tour de France.

THE TOUR RACE RADIO CRACKLED.

'Chute, chute!'

Always in French. No emotion. *'Chute, chute!'*

Meaning 'crash'.

Right away the atmosphere in the car changed. We held our breath, waiting to hear who was involved. Was it our . . .?

'Team Sky. Team Sky.'

It was.

With me in the car was the *directeur sportif,* Sean Yates, and a mechanic, Diego Costa. Yates was driving, his hand jammed on the horn as the Jaguar surged forward, towards the scene of the crash. Diego and I gathered our stuff. We knew what to do; we'd been in this situation enough times for it to be routine.

In the pre-stage team talk on the Team Sky bus – the 'Death Star' – Yates had highlighted this section of the race as a 'heads up' moment, when, after a long flat straight, the road turned acutely and narrowed. It was a perfect place for a rival to launch an attack as the peloton – that's the main group of cyclists, each one a centimetre from his neighbour – slowed and backed up.

The potential for a crash was huge.

Sure enough . . .

The Jag screamed to a halt and we bundled out like troops deploying from an army helicopter: me clutching my trauma bag; Diego with a front and rear bike wheel, the two of us sprinting along a sun-dappled road in search of our fallen comrades.

The road was dry and there were plenty of skid marks, which was encouraging. It meant there had been time to brake, slow down and lose momentum before the big bang.

And there he was, Bradley Wiggins, sitting with his head down – a good sign, in that he was conscious and breathing – amid a scene of general carnage, riders and bikes everywhere.

But everyone was moving.

It's when they're not moving. That's when it's bad. That's when you really worry.

I looked into Wiggins's eyes. The lights were on. My first duty after establishing that the patient is breathing, his heart is beating and he's not bleeding profusely (and Wiggins was conscious, cursing, and there was no pool of blood) is to clear the neck. Cervical spine trauma can damage the spinal cord and can mean permanent paralysis. All good there.

Next, no overt concussion.

Now my hands swept gently over his clavicle. For a cyclist fracturing the clavicle is the most common injury. I knew what I was going to find.

It was broken.

He tried to get up. I told him to stay down.

He got up anyway. Diego offered him a spare bike and he tried to take hold of it, failed and let fly with a fresh torrent of swear words.

Meanwhile, the rest of the team were waiting, waiting to assist Wiggins back into the race, which had disappeared over the horizon. I yelled at them that he was out and slowly, reluctantly, they drifted off, back to the peloton.

Moments later, the Team Sky Jaguar pushed past, and they instinctively regrouped, adjusting to a new set of priorities, Yates giving me a short nod as he passed. There's little room for sentiment on the Tour de France. Besides, Yates had prepared all season for this, his twenty-first Tour.

Not for the first time I was left behind with an injured rider, and

I helped him to the waiting ambulance, the wailing siren clearing a route through the crowds of spectators, cars and motorhomes.

The rest was routine. A visit to the hospital. Examination. His road rash cleaned and dressed. I did it myself with the help of a nurse, the casualty doctor observing and asking about the race – a fan, as it turned out.

We left as soon as we could, trading a Team Sky racing jersey for a disc of X-ray images and stepping out into the car park. A TV reporter was waiting, and Wiggins started talking, his tongue loosened by morphine, a string of unbroadcastable bad language.

The long and the short of it was that he was out of that year's Tour de France.

I'd already spoken to the orthopaedic surgeon. Surgery was scheduled for the next day. Wiggins, meanwhile, would have to deal with his disappointment and concentrate on the following year's Tour de France.

Perhaps 2012 would be his year.

Wiggins was our GC, which means the general classification rider – our top man, in other words. The team had pinned its hopes on him winning the Tour de France, and it was up to me as the team's doctor to make sure he was in the right shape to do so.

It was the same with every athlete on our riding staff. While it was up to the coaches to train the riders, it was my responsibility – and that of the doctors in my charge – to ensure they were in the right shape to be trained, to help them stay in that condition and then patch them up if and when things went wrong.

This book is all about that process. It's about how I took a background in sports science, honed in professional football, and applied it to cycling, where it helped power success in the 2012 London Olympics and the Tour de France in the same year – to name but two of many sporting triumphs. It's about the medical issues particular to cyclists and what we do about them; it's about the mindset of the rider and how that feeds into the physical side of what they do.

Needless to say, we'll go behind the scenes at British Cycling and Team Sky in order to touch upon the issues unique to those teams, where the pressure on riders and coaches to perform meant that I often found myself performing a delicate balancing act whilst protecting athlete welfare (because the fact is that sport isn't always healthy, and there are risks associated with athletes needing to train when ill or injured). I'll talk about the difficulty of trying to find the balance between medicine and sport, the watchfulness required to ensure that sport is not in thrall to medicine, and that it's never a case of allowing the tail to wag the dog. And we'll discuss the business of risk-managing patients both in the short and long term, and how these two remits can so often come into conflict.

In addition to all of that I hope there's plenty in here that will prove informative, helpful, even inspirational for the amateur cyclist, because while the focus is on my work with the likes of Bradley Wiggins, Chris Hoy, Victoria Pendleton *et al*, it's also about the issues relevant to all cyclists; and how you as an enthusiast can improve your overall health, not just in cycling but in your day-to-day life.

Moreover, it's about the line. The start. The finish. Finding it. Making others aware of it. Going up to it.

But never crossing it.

1

A Day in the Life (part one)

The beginning of a typical day with Team Sky, from waking up to breakfast time, meeting the team and learning how sports medicine plays a vital part in what we do . . .

WHETHER AT TRAINING CAMP or on tour, a rider's day is structured similarly and always starts with a pee into a pot. If they're lucky they might be able to do it without someone else watching. For a rider, that's a good day.

Training or tour, breakfast is usually around 8am, but most people in the camp will have been up since around six, apart from the mechanics, who often work through the night and so tend to rise a little later. The team principal, Dave Brailsford, and the coaches all go for a group ride before breakfast on their state-of-the-art, race-prepared Pinarellos – two hours' cycling, without fail (Sean Yates would do a six-hour stint). Whether we're at camp or on tour, they always do it.

If it's a race day, the *soigneurs* get up at the crack of dawn. The *soigneurs* are the assistants who are first and foremost soft-tissue masseurs but also work as general gofers ('*soigneur*' translates as 'the one who provides care'), and it's their job to prepare the in-race food and drinks filled with electrolytes and carbohydrates. Everybody on a race team works hard. None more so than the *soigneurs* – or 'swannies' as they tend to be called.

Meanwhile, the riders get up moments before breakfast, savouring every last minute of rest before shuffling slowly to my room, which is converted into a makeshift medical quarters for the duration of our stay. When I say 'shuffle', I mean it, because whenever a rider is not on a bike he or she is conserving energy. They never stand when they can sit; they never take the stairs if there's a lift available; they never sit if they can lie down; they never carry anything if there's a *soigneur* to carry it for them. Our British Cycling riders were absent from the Grand Opening of the 2012 Olympics. Why? Because we were a performance-driven team and Brailsford wasn't going to have people standing around for three hours when they could be on their bed resting.

So anyway, that's start of my morning. A stream of bleary-eyed riders. They come for urine-concentration testing, weight testing, and to get the third degree from me.

'How are you feeling?'

'All right. Yeah. Good. Great.'

'How did you sleep?'

'Head on the pillow. Usual way, Doc, you know.'

Wiggins is a great mimic, and with me being from Lancashire he takes enormous delight in impersonating my accent. It's one of the ways I can tell if he's all right or not, which is generally the point of the morning inquisition: how do you feel it went yesterday? Any excessive fatigue? Do you have any significant muscle soreness? How's the saddle sore, the road rash? Geraint Thomas would usually promise me some of his mother's Welsh cakes for the race car. If he didn't, I knew to ask more questions.

As their doctor I'm trying to find out if they're over-exerting, over-stressing or under-recovering. In short, I need to know if they're on it or off it. The questions, they are what they are. The replies might be truthful, considered or flippant. It doesn't really matter. Most of the time I can tell just by looking in their eyes.

Off they go, leaving me alone to analyse their urine and cross-reference their weight stats.

Now, if we're on tour, we might be subject to a dawn raid from the anti-doping people, who will knock on my door, give me a list of two to four riders they want to see, and I'll have to go and wake the riders up.

'Don't have a pee, testers are here,' I'd tell the riders.

That's crucial, the not-having-a-pee. If they have a pee then they're waiting maybe two hours to get enough urine into their bladder in order to give a 90ml sample, and you ain't going nowhere until you've given that sample, because if you don't provide a sample then it's an anti-doping rule violation, a strike, and you only get three of those in twelve months before a one to two-year sanction. It's not the strike we worry about so much as the reputation damage. So, if a rider can't provide his urine in the morning and the bus is leaving at nine o'clock, they get left behind until they can.

So, not exactly an ideal way for an athlete to start his day, but I will say this: not once was any rider unpleasant or rude to the doping control staff, no matter how tired they were, or how early it was. To them, it's just part of the job. The company most often sent by the UCI (the Union Cycliste Internationale – the world governing body of the sport) to test us was Clearidium. Wiggins called them 'chlamydia' and the name stuck.

A chaperone goes into the toilet with the rider who must be naked from the nipples to the knees – full exposure, in other words, to prevent someone using a bag and tube catheter to give another person's urine. The chaperone will watch the rider peeing – he must be able to see the end of the urethra – into the sterile collection pot. The rider – always the rider – then divides it into an 'A' sample, which is analysed at an accredited laboratory, usually within days, and a 'B' sample, which is sent off and frozen. If there's an adverse analytical finding in the A sample, potentially a drug infringement, something banned under the WADA (World Anti-Doping Agency) code, the team is allowed to have the B sample analysed and a team doctor witness it, to ensure it's a proper analysis. Thankfully, this never happened on my watch.

Athletes are invited to list their medications, although it's not compulsory. Some list them in minute detail. One British Cycling rider used to ask for a supplementary piece of paper for her list of drugs, medications, supplements and homeopathic remedies.

But anyway, if the testers don't come then the riders can pee how and when they like – so long as I get my sample. While I'm in my room surrounded by their urine, they will take the lift to the dining room, where pride of place at the centre of each table is a large dispenser of hand sanitiser.

The hand sanitiser represents what Team Sky, and 'marginal gains', is all about.

Planning for the Tour de France starts in October, when the following year's route is announced. But in a way, we're always preparing for the Tour de France for the simple reason that it's cycling's biggest race, has the greatest prestige and is the prize that our team principal, Brailsford, sets his sights on winning.

The concept of 'marginal gains' is key to Brailsford's strategy. It's a concept widely thought to be his brainchild, although I believe that the origins of these practices can be seen in other arenas (which we'll come to). Either way, it was Brailsford who perfected it. No doubt he named it, too.

The principle of marginal gains means making small improvements in all aspects of the team process in order to create one overall performance advantage. It involves looking at every single thing we do, from coaching to catering to my own speciality, sports medicine, and asking how we can refine and improve it: what small, incremental adjustments can we make that, while tiny themselves, will give us the edge?

Hence the fact that wherever we are in the world, whatever the competition, whatever we're doing at any given time, pride of place at the centre of the table is always a large bottle of hand sanitiser. Minimising the spread of infection falls squarely within the remit of marginal gains.

I'd come from Bolton Wanderers, where we weren't as obsessive about the risk of minor infections, partly because staying infection free isn't as crucial to a football player as it is to a rider, and partly because football's a team sport. There are places to hide. You can be below your best and still function as part of a winning team.

Not so for riders. In cycling, athletes are at the peak of aerobic and anaerobic performance. They have to be almost one hundred per cent fit all of the time, otherwise they'll get left behind. 'Dropped', in cycling parlance.

So in cycling there is no such thing as a minor infection. A footballer, even if not operating at their personal best, can still turn a game with that long ball. A golfer with a sore throat is capable of a jaw-dropping putt. But there is no such thing as a great rider below peak fitness. Their talent is so closely linked to their fitness as to be indiscernible from it.

They're odd people. Obsessed by numbers, power output, the miles they've done, the metres they've climbed, their pedalling cadence (pedal rotation speed), their heart rate, their weight, the bike's weight, their gear ratios, and any other numbers you care to put in front of them. In the Premiership, a player will do anything to get out of training, but just try keeping a rider off their bike. Even during the off season they'll go out every day, just to do what they call 'spinning their legs'. They like their own company, they love pushing themselves – I believe they might actually enjoy suffering – and they train and train and train in order to extract the best performance from their body.

I'll give you an example of just how deep their dedication is. After that crash in 2011, Wiggins had surgery on his clavicle.

A Day in the Life (part one)

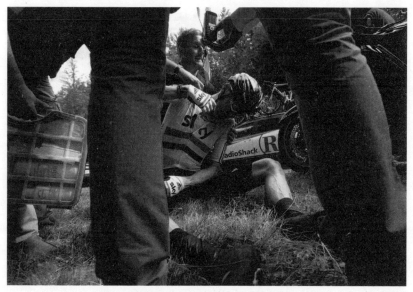

Bradley Wiggins fractures his left collar bone,
stage 7, 2011 Tour de France.

Now, normally if you fracture your clavicle and get it fixed on the NHS, they won't plate it because it's expensive and will heal fine in a sling. Is the result as good? No. I know an orthopaedic surgeon. He broke his clavicle. What did he do? He had it plated. But that's another story.

So we flew Bradley Wiggins back from France and the clavicle was plated in Manchester. But the plating doesn't provide any strength in the clavicle, it just puts the two ends together and immobilises it so that they can heal as rapidly possible and in the correct alignment needed for athletic performance. Ultimately the plate does nothing for strength, it's the bone-to-bone healing that's important, and the bone won't be strong for up to twelve weeks.

But Wiggins was back training for the Vuelta a España, the grand tour of Spain, three days after the op.

Riders use an indoor cycling simulator called a turbo trainer. They slot their bikes into it and it allows them to train stationary. They love it because when it's pouring down with rain or icy outside they can put on their headphones and ride a bike in their garage for hours on end.

I've seen injured riders training at the velodrome bring in their bike and set up a turbo in the gym. I'd go away, forget about them and then realise it had been four hours since I'd seen them; I'd go back in and they'd still be there, whirring away.

Wiggins was back in his turbo trainer three days after his operation, totally dedicated. Absolutely on it.

We also had a horse treadmill at the velodrome, which allows a rider to alter the speed and gradient of the climb while being supported by a harness so if he fell off he didn't crash and get swept back by the treadmill. He was soon on that, too.

And if this is an example of how committed – if occasionally almost masochistic – riders are, it also works as an example of the way that we practised performance health management in professional sports at Team Sky. I like to think of it as 'performance medicine'. He was on morphine, which affects a patient's psychomotor coordination; he would have been a danger if we'd let him out on the road, as another fall this early would almost certainly break the plated clavicle again.

In this situation, the two disciplines – medicine and sport – worked together, tailored to help maintain his fitness as well playing an important psychological role.

A Day in the Life (part one)

Medicine taps into the cyclist's need for control over their training programme, which is closely linked to their fear of the random variable. It's why medicine has come to play such an important part in sport over recent years, because it can help control the uncontrollable.

Can it, though? Can it really? It doesn't matter. The important thing is that medicine is perceived to help control the uncontrollable, and that in itself creates a huge psychological advantage. During this book we'll talk about 'the placebo effect', where a treatment of some kind – and it doesn't have to be a drug, it could be a supplement or support bandage, anything – produces a beneficial effect which has nothing to do with the treatment itself and everything to do with the patient's belief in the treatment; we'll talk about the doctor-as-talisman: to what extent the benefits of my presence and the treatment I administered were in fact wrapped up in the psychology of an athlete. But that doesn't mean it's all snake oil, far from it. The fact is, a doctor can help – or as I say, be perceived to help, which amounts to the same thing – in controlling the uncontrollable, alleviating the rider's fear of the random.

All of which brings us back to the hand sanitiser. Because there's nothing more random than an infection.

To you and me an upper respiratory tract infection is a sniffle, a cold. You're blowing your nose and feeling a bit under the weather. To a rider it's the difference between tenth place and first.

Gastroenteritis to you and me means the trots and making sure you're never too far from a toilet. To a rider it means they're not absorbing nutrients efficiently, they're losing electrolytes. Or, worse, they're becoming dehydrated. All of which is crippling for an athlete's performance.

We cut down on infections such as these once we introduced the hand sanitiser. And it wasn't all in the minds of the riders. We really did, because you're just as likely to get an upper respiratory tract infection or gastroenteritis from shaking hands with somebody who's infected, as being sneezed on or eating food prepared by them. We also attempted to introduce a no-hand-shaking rule, as we had done at Bolton, where Sam Allardyce discouraged the morning ritual of shaking literally everyone's hand on arrival at the players' and staff lounge at the training ground. Whenever I saw anybody who looked even slightly unwell, they were either asked to stay away or I gave them one of the small travel-sized bottles of hand sanitiser I used to carry around with me specifically for that purpose.

We also introduced a policy of always closing the toilet lid whenever anyone flushed the toilet. If there's infection in the toilet, which is highly likely, and you flush it with the lid open, you create an aerosol effect, and even if you've exited the bathroom or cubicle by the time that happens, you risk getting it on your toothbrush, say, so the next time you brush your teeth you can pick up the infection.

We made ourselves unpopular sometimes. Myself and the team nutritionist, Nigel Mitchell, would inspect hotel kitchens, and if we didn't like the standard of hygiene then changes would have to be made. On one occasion we even moved hotel. Later we'd take our own chef on tour, and ultimately we had our own catering truck in order to have complete control over the hygiene of what the athletes ate.

Back to my room, then, and one of the key reasons I'm in there analysing the riders' urine and weight. Twice daily, weight is studied to learn how much fluid has been lost, rather than trying to assess loss of muscle mass. Changes in urine concentration are also used to determine hydration status. Armed with the facts I join the riders at breakfast, going from table to table with the results: yes, it's good; no, it's bad, you need to drink more. With effective on-bike feeding and refuelling before and after racing we hoped to maintain the rider's weight throughout a Grand Tour, and usually managed it, saving the rider's body from searching for missing calories by metabolising their own muscles for energy.

It's an uphill battle getting them to drink their two litres of fruit juice and water mixture before training or on their way to the race, but I stick with it. The idea is that they're almost over-hydrated by the time they get to the start line, because hydration is hugely important to what we do. We've performed sweat analysis in order to tailor rehydration to the individual but it proved logistically impossible to do whilst racing. So it's plain water, or water with electrolytes, sometimes with carbohydrate. Whatever mixture we use, it's always fluid taken orally. Historically, cycling has used intravenous fluids to rehydrate athletes but that's unnecessary unless you're ill, suffering from something like gastroenteritis, in which case you'd be in a clinic, not racing. Besides, you have eighteen hours before racing starts again. That's eighteen hours to orally rehydrate an athlete, which is more than ample.

Breakfast is the most important meal of the day and they use it to load up on protein and carbohydrates. For protein it's eggs, scrambled or an omelette, however they like it, and a lot of eggs, too, as well as yoghurt – another good protein source – with fruit. For carbohydrates it's typically porridge with agave syrup. There's always a lot of coffee.

It's a chatty, social time, unlike the evening meals, when athletes are tired and mulling over the day's work, and they'll be talking about whatever riders talk about, which is cycling. Riders are absolutely consumed with cycling. For most of them it's the way they engage with the world. Meanwhile, the coaches and management are discussing strategies, confirming which are the key climbs, which riders and teams are threats, how the race will be controlled. It really is a team sport, something I had not truly grasped as a Tour de France armchair viewer.

The race programme for the Grand Tour GC contender is chosen carefully. Particular races have more importance for sponsors and the team will target those more aggressively than others. There are well-known preparation races – the Critérium du Dauphiné, the Tour de Romandie – which not only give a comparative test to GC competitors but assess form for the Tour de France, which again is key, because sport is all about form. You can be as well prepared as possible, but unless you have that magical thing called form – and it doesn't matter whether you're playing football, golf or cycling – you're lost.

Still, none of this is really my domain. I love sports, I love medicine, and I really love sports medicine, but my primary philosophy is one of 'do no harm'. I'm particularly keen to discourage the 'winning at all costs' mentality that has a habit of creeping into professional sport.

My concern is for the athletes. They're patients first, riders second.

2

A Sports Medic is Born

The beginnings of my medical life, embracing the 'new' discipline of sports science en route to British Cycling and Team Sky, and gaining an understanding of some of the issues at play

I WAS RAISED IN GATLEY, MANCHESTER. My dad was a vet, my mum was a radiographer, my uncle was a doctor and, subsequently, my younger brother became a doctor, too.

It was hardly a surprise, then, that I went from Manchester Grammar School to Cambridge University and then on to Manchester Medical School.

I loved medical school. I enjoyed student lifestyle free of financial responsibility, but most of all I loved studying, learning. I was like a sponge, and in many ways I've never really stopped being a sponge. It's one of the reasons that medicine has never lost its fascination for me. There's always something new to learn about.

As for what I'd do after medical school? Well, for a short period I quite liked the idea of anaesthetics. But then I went off the idea when somebody warned me that I'd spend most of my time monitoring an anaesthetised patient's vital signs. And your patients can't talk. In other words, it could be very dull indeed.

Instead I found myself looking in the direction of general practice and after leaving hospital training I joined a practice in Whalley, Lancashire, as a trainee, and then was invited to stay on as a partner. There, we looked after a local maternity hospital and a local cottage hospital, and we had our own pharmacy as well. It was great, not just because I loved and still do love Whalley, in the glorious Ribble Valley, but also because it was the days of proper, *personal* doctoring, which suited me down to the ground. If I had entered medicine with a fascination for learning, then I stayed because of a fascination for people. And while some GPs can be very abrupt – 'Here's what's wrong with you, here's what to take. Next!' – I found myself taking a more holistic approach, really listening and doing my best to get to the root of the underlying, often hidden, problem.

As you might imagine, there's a time cost involved; I was always a doctor to run late in surgery, while at the same time I started to attract those who needed my sort of approach, the type of patient whose problems had emotional and psychological elements – family disharmony and the like. So not only was it time-consuming but it was emotionally demanding as well.

I was already married by then. I'd met Frankie when I was sixteen. I became a medical student and she chose nursing and we married in 1982. I qualified in 1984. We already had four kids under five by the time I ended up in Whalley, so it was hard work for us both. Rewarding. But hard. Hard enough that, in 1990, after six years, feeling emotionally drained and exhausted and wanting to do something different, I found myself on a two-day residential course in sports medicine at Lilleshall, run by the British Association of Sport and Exercise Medicine – the first course of its kind. It was a combination of my two great interests, sport and medicine, a new discipline to learn. I was instantly smitten.

Around the same time I met a guy who had been a GP then trained as an osteopath, and had become what was known as a musculoskeletal physician. Talking to him I found that I liked the idea of osteopathy, with its emphasis on musculoskeletal symptoms. Traditional doctors tend to rely a lot more on imaging and medication, whereas osteopaths assess and treat the tissues with their hands, and I saw this as potentially an additional way of making my musculoskeletal diagnoses.

Next I took leave to study for an MSc in Musculoskeletal Medicine, which included a year at an osteopathic college in London, and meant leaving full-time general practice in Whalley and job sharing with a colleague from medical school at a practice down the road in Clitheroe. At the same time, I started a clinic in the practice for musculoskeletal problems, running it alongside studying for my diploma in sports medicine.

Part-time jobs in sport followed. For a while I was doctor on the European Golf Tour, the highlight being when the European Team won the Ryder Cup at the Belfry in 2002. I also worked as an assistant at Burnley football club, after which I was paid to get involved with the FA, who wanted a medical presence on their inaugural doping control programme. I provided medical cover at a World Rally Championship, and went to Cyprus with the Ford Motor Sport team.

At the same time, I founded an NHS musculoskeletal medicine service in East Lancashire where we employed physiotherapists and other doctors to treat patients with musculoskeletal conditions that didn't require surgery. What sort of conditions? Say, for example, a patient presented with tennis elbow that had been unresponsive to the usual treatment of rest, massage and ibuprofen, we'd start with eccentric strengthening exercises, which work by exercising the muscles the wrong way round so they lengthen during contraction when they usually shorten. It seems wrong and it's painful and patients need to be given the confidence and reassurance to do it. Some would need injection therapy.

At the musculoskeletal medicine service, we invested £60,000 on a diagnostic ultrasound machine which used sound waves to create an image of inside the body. It was a revelation, helping with diagnosis and also to guide injections accurately and safely.

I was working there when I got the call to help out at Bolton Wanderers Football Club – mainly evening and weekend cover – while the usual doctor went off to do some cover at the Rugby Five Nations. There I got to meet a hugely important figure in my career: Bolton's then-manager, Sam Allardyce.

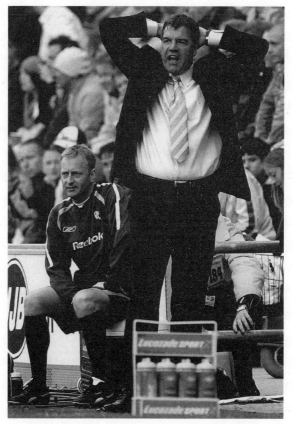

Sam Allardyce, manager Bolton Wanderers FC;
seated is Mark Taylor, his right-hand man.

'One thing you've got to remember, Doc,' he said to me. 'All players are see-you-next-Tuesdays.'

It took me a second to work out what he meant, but I got there.

'And as long as you don't let them get between us we'll be fine.'

The temporary position led to a permanent job as team doctor, my first full-time job in sports, and it was there at Bolton that

I learnt what it was that I really loved about sports medicine. I was dealing with patients who were highly motivated, stretching their bodies to the limit, adapting and improving; anatomy, physiology and psychology; high performance not deterioration and death.

Another thing, of course, was the resources. Back in those days there would have been an eighteen-month waiting list for an MR scan of a lumbar spine problem on the NHS. In sports medicine you requested a scan and two hours later the scan would be taking place.

At Bolton we always had slots reserved at a private hospital for after a match so we could just phone up and the players would waltz in. The hospital had the prestige of being associated with the club – they'd get a signed shirt for reception – and as a result they went the extra mile for us.

Later, at British Cycling and Team Sky, we had use of the MR scanner installed on the premises at the Manchester Institute of Health & Performance, a building funded by Manchester City Football Club in conjunction with the local council. Less than 500 metres as the crow flies.

Speaking purely as a sports doctor, it was just about perfect. If you or I have a sore knee, we don't get an MR scan that day. Or that month. But if you're an athlete, you do. The immediacy of the process was incredibly attractive to me.

Not only that, but scans were electronically transmitted from the hospital to me, so I could see the results seconds after they'd taken place. I could then send the results to anyone I wanted to read them, which was usually Dr Phil O'Connor, a consultant musculoskeletal radiologist from the Leeds Teaching Hospitals (who went on to run the imaging centre at London 2012), and *the* person to discuss an athlete's scan with.

Wherever in the world we went, if I did a scan, an X-ray, whatever, I'd send it electronically for his opinion. It became a thing for him: Friday night in his kitchen in Leeds, reading Doc Freeman's scans.

And then there was Sam Allardyce.

There's a reason he's called Big Sam. He's big in physical appearance, big presence and big personality. Not only that, but he's a very intelligent bloke. He could see things – he knew what was coming, what was just around the corner – and that's why he was one of the first managers in the Premiership to embrace sports science. Things that sound simple now – I'm talking really basic stuff, like putting electrolytes in sports drinks – he adopted at a time when most teams were still serving their players tea from an urn.

He and I hit it off professionally for that reason. Previous doctors at Bolton had been jobbing GPs, doctors who liked sport, whose job was fire-fighting, patching up players when they got hurt.

I brought something new to the table – sports medicine – which was all about being proactive, about preparing players and helping them to recover properly from exertion and injury.

The physiotherapist at Bolton was an ex-professional footballer, Mark Taylor. When his career ended in injury he studied for a degree in sports science and then a degree in physiotherapy. He obviously knew his sport, the demands and the health issues that were important. He embraced prevention and innovation quite naturally. Between us, we practised a form of medicine known as 'performance health management' – by which I mean that we pledged to find the right ethical and operational balance between health *management* and optimising *performance*. We were adherents of sport-specific training, physiotherapy, strength and conditioning, nutrition, hydration and recovery. We emphasised the importance of core stability, strength and flexibility, which meant that instead of training for two hours and then going off to play golf, players had to spend time in the gym, working on their core. We were among the first, if not *the* first, to put theory into practice.

Which brings me back to a point I made earlier, because I think it was Sam Allardyce who was in fact the innovator of what became known as marginal gains. Because although he may not have given it a title, or even adopted it as a formal philosophy, he certainly believed in it. It was just part of his management style. He was all about getting the basics right in order to make overall improvements.

It's one of the reasons that during Sam's time with Bolton the team punched above its weight. Another reason was that he could see that some players who had fallen off the conveyor belt, often due to psychological problems, sometimes for physical reasons, were hidden gems. And he brought them back, making them great players again.

Allardyce was also a proponent of yoga and a supporter of using performance analysis statistics. He was a huge believer in preparation and recovery, and was absolutely committed to many of the practices that, with his help, I introduced to the club.

For instance, he had read somewhere that tooth fillings – aka 'dental amalgams' – at least the mercury-based ones, were bad for you, so he said, 'Right, get all these fuckers in here, they're all going to have their fillings out,' and the players loved it because they were replacing unsightly mercury-based fillings with more natural-looking white ceramic ones. They extended it to staff, too. I did it. Allardyce did it. We had all our old fillings taken out and ceramic ones put in.

Not everything we did was a success, but most of it was, and I count myself very lucky to have worked with Allardyce so early on. If I'd come up against a manager with a more, shall we say, 'traditional' approach to sports science, then I'm certain I would have been banging my head against a brick wall.

Mind you, he was still an 'old skool' gaffer in many ways, and I remember old and new coming into contact after one particular match when he thought the players had underperformed. We'd introduced a policy for the players of eating trendy antioxidant 'super fruits' after a game. Again, this was a time when players would have preferred to go for a pint and pie rather than eat fruit, but we were in the vanguard of trying to change that attitude, and so we had bowls of blueberries for them to graze on (grazing: very important for the athlete).

These bowls of blueberries were on the table as Allardyce was giving his players both barrels, disgusted at their performance. In a fit of anger, he slammed his fist down and sent blueberries flying everywhere. Antioxidant super fruit lost out to good old English football management on that occasion.

That was him all over. We used to run a sweepstake: how many times would Sam use the F-word in his post-match talk?

One of his particular success stories was the player Gary Speed, who played until he was thirty-seven, quite an age for a professional football player. Speed's fitness levels were remarkable, and that's because he looked after himself. He understood the importance of diet, recovery and sleep, as well as the deleterious effects of alcohol on the athletic body and mind. He embraced ice baths, whole body cryotherapy, post-exercise protein and rehydration. And because he was so well respected by the players, he was a real cheerleader for some of the more progressive practices.

Speed was also one of those rare people who are just genetically well made to endure the particular rigours of professional sport. This usually means that they don't seem to suffer the musculo-skeletal injuries, tendinopathies and articular cartilage problems that other athletes do, that compromise their careers.

All in all, he was a great player, and a great man, and I was very distressed to hear of his suicide in 2011. Naturally I thought, 'Were there signs that could have been spotted?'

I'm sure everyone who has any association with suicide goes through those same feelings.

But although Speed and I had a good relationship, I was never really friends with him. And it was always the same throughout my entire career, whether it was football, golf, cycling or in general practice. I never went to retirement parties or weddings. I never tried to be a friend. I was never a fan. I tried to practise a policy of never having a favourite.

* * *

A Sports Medic is Born

Back to Bolton, and Allardyce resigned in April 2007, which was a huge blow for me personally and professionally because I did not feel his replacements were quite so progressive when it came to sports science. I handed in my notice and went back into clinical medicine at the NHS, thinking that perhaps my days as a team doctor were over.

Not so. There I was one afternoon when the phone rang and I found myself talking to Dave Brailsford's assistant, Fran Millar.

A new road cycling team, Team Sky, was looking for doctors, she told me. Would I be interested?

Prior to that call, my interest in cycling was restricted to watching the Tour de France on TV. At that point I had no idea that it was effectively a last-man-standing race, which is not something I can wholeheartedly support as a doctor, but it looked exciting. It also hadn't escaped my notice that British cyclists had been doing well at the Olympics. I was intrigued enough to meet Brailsford.

He turned out to be a fascinating bloke. A dome-headed, forceful, inspiring character, he was a cycling enthusiast who'd left the small town in North Wales in which he'd grown up in order to try and make it as a professional rider in Europe. He became a *soigneur* in professional cycling before rising – or should that be riding – up the ranks and then, to cut a long story short, he ended up as performance director of British Cycling, which was on its knees at the time.

Brailsford, the head coach Shane Sutton and the then head of medicine Dr Steve Peters, had turned it all around. They had made British Cycling 'the medal factory'. They were the untouchables.

31

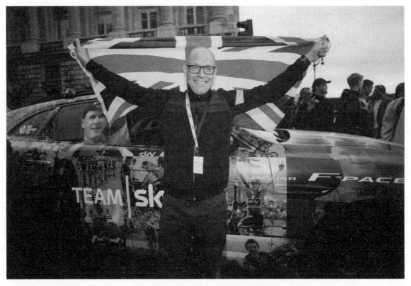

Sir Dave Brailsford. Architect of the greatest revolution
in British sporting history.

As I say, Brailsford himself is a passionate cyclist, in great
physical condition. I did a medical on him last year and he's got
the body fat percentage and cardiovascular function of an elite
athlete. Even though the track was his bread and butter, and
where the medals were coming from, his heart lay in road racing.

Thus, after a terrific showing at the Beijing Olympics in 2008
– fourteen medals, domination in road and track – Brailsford
had decided he wanted to form a pro-tour team – a road team
that could race the Tour de France.

He went in search of backing and found it in the shape of
Rupert Murdoch's son James, another cycling enthusiast, who put
money into the team, now Team Sky. Brailsford began recruiting
staff and coaches, and then cyclists, keeping the emphasis on

British personnel and shying away from anybody with a history of doping.

'We'll never cross that blue line,' was one of his favourite sayings. 'I'll never ask you to cross it.'

The literal 'blue line' to which he referred was the one that ran around the velodrome track, below which was reserved for racing. But for Brailsford, and indeed all of us at British Cycling and Team Sky, it also represented an ethical line we had pledged not to cross. We were going to win fair and square.

We would never cheat.

Cycling, of course, had a long and dishonourable history in that regard. Mechanical cheating was not unknown, but by far the biggest area of deception was 'doping' – using prohibited drugs to enhance performance – with Lance Armstrong and the Festina team being the most high-profile but by no means only offenders. The sport was just emerging from an era when mass doping amongst riders was not only commonplace but actually encouraged by the teams. You were considered to be letting the side down if you didn't do it.

The most common substance to be used – indeed, the drug that Lance Armstrong had abused for years, injected by the now-disgraced doctor Michele Ferrari – was EPO (otherwise known as Erythropoietin), a performance-enhancing drug that stimulates the bone marrow to produce new red blood cells, basically boosting the oxygen-carrying capacity of blood. It had been banned since the early 1990s, and was undetectable until the year 2000.

It was EPO that David Millar of Great Britain was busted for possessing in 2004, at which point he admitted to having used it since 2001. Millar – the brother of Team Sky's Fran, who had phoned me that day – has since become something of an anti-doping spokesman, which is fair enough and entirely admirable, but for the fact that he had a lot to say in the wake of the news that Wiggins had been injected with triamcinolone, suggesting in a *New York Times* article, 'How to Get Away With Doping', that triamcinolone had performance-enhancing properties.

Wiggins had indeed been injected with medical doses of triamcinolone under a TUE, which is a 'therapeutic use exemption' allowed under the WADA code. But if triamcinolone had performance-enhancing capabilities, it would not be allowed by WADA, even under a TUE.

It's a subject that we will, of course, return to.

Back to Brailsford, then, and like Allardyce he was a bit . . . different. There was just something about him. A charisma. A focus. A clear sense of mission. Also like Allardyce he was capable of inspiring those around him.

It's no surprise the two men were fundamentally similar. They moved in a lot of the same circles. Both Brailsford and Allardyce would attend think tanks that the former Arsenal manager Arsène Wenger conducted at his home. And they also shared – crucially, where I was concerned – an interest in sports medicine.

'Listen,' Brailsford told me. 'I'm looking for doctors with a skill set. I don't want a GP who likes sport. I don't want a cycling fan who fancies getting closer to the action. I want someone who's into sports medicine, who can help us win the Tour de France within five years, and do it clean.'

3

A Clean Sheet

*The realities of life at Team Sky, and the duty of
care I owed my new patients*

I WAS, TO ALL INTENTS AND PURPOSES, the doctor to all of
the athletes, taking the place of their usual physician. There were
twenty-nine riders at Team Sky, and then a further hundred at
British Cycling. Clearly, there was a lot of overlap between the
two, not least because we shared headquarters at the Manchester
velodrome and a team principal. But without doubt Team Sky
was the shining star. If you were in Team Sky, you'd get the iMac,
iPhone, smarter training shoes and posh suitcases, as well as use
of the team car, a sponsored Jaguar. As you might imagine, it
created something of a division, even a little jealousy between the
two teams.

As far as I was concerned, it was often a challenge to keep
the two strands separate, but the main difference between the

two was their gender make-up. Team Sky's riding staff were all male, whereas the split was closer to half-and-half at British Cycling.

Brailsford came in for a lot of criticism for Team Sky's exclusion of women, and understandably so. To my mind having a women's team was a no-brainer and could have helped increase coverage in women's racing, as well as decreasing the existing gender pay gap (a gap that thanks to the work of athletes such as Lizzie Deignan is slowly being closed).

There are those who say that men's races are more exciting, but as someone who enjoys women's football, I disagree. I was once the medical officer at the Women's Euro and I saw talented, athletic, competitive players with a huge buzz and a passion for the game. I also sensed a belief in equality, and it was incredibly refreshing.

That aside, the operation at Team Sky was truly impressive. It was as much a worldwide logistics company as it was a bike team. I was based at the Manchester velodrome, but the riders lived throughout Europe. Our operations centre, called the service course, where the bikes and equipment were stored and where the mechanics were based when not on tour was in Belgium in a town called Deinze in Flanders.

In addition there was a car park where the two Death Star tour buses – they were commonly known as Death Stars because of their distinctive look – were kept, as well as three air-conditioned mechanics' trucks. (Air-conditioned, because everybody works better when it's 21 degrees than when it's 40. Mechanics are no different. It wasn't luxury, just another marginal gain.)

There was no specific training base for Team Sky. For them the December–January training camp in Majorca, or the high altitude of Mount Teide in Tenerife was when they got together to train as a team.

The Team Sky riders being so spread out made it something of a challenge to look after them, much more so than British Cycling riders, who were based in the same place that they trained, with medical facilities nearby. Often, Team Sky riders would be assessed at races and then brought back to Manchester if they had a medical issue.

Sometimes they'd stay in their location – Gerona and Nice, places like that – and a member of the medical staff would then be despatched to see them, or we'd have a trusted colleague in the private sector take a look at them.

Meanwhile British Cycling riders trained at the velodrome, where they'd have priority over the public, although the coaches still had to reserve and pay for track time. Also in the velodrome were my offices and medical facilities which, as I soon discovered, were a little on the basic side, certainly compared to what I'd been used to at Bolton.

A velodrome consists of a concrete base laid with wooden track. In Manchester it was Siberian spruce and proved to be very fast. My room was basically built into the foundations of the track. I used to be able to hear the riders going round and round above my head, an almost hypnotic drumming sound that came to soundtrack my days there.

The carpet. Ugh. It was microbiologically disgusting and medically unacceptable. Almost the first thing I did was to get it removed and vinyl floor that could be cleaned with antiseptic was put down.

It had a very basic sink, no taps that could be closed with elbows when scrubbing up to suture as in general practice. If I wanted a rider to pass a specimen of urine, they had to go all the way down the corridor to the track toilet used by the public and then bring it back. Not only that, but the walls and door had little soundproofing and no lockable pharmaceutical store. These were issues that I had to deal with as a matter of some urgency, and it took a while but I did eventually get the funding to buy lockable medicine cupboards in which to store my drugs.

As for my travelling kit, I used to take a massive holdall, two feet wide and eighteen inches tall, full of medicines, camomile tea, Fisherman's Friend lozenges (more on those later), hand sanitiser and plastic bags for vomit (more on those later, too).

My holdall would go on tour with us. It was like my toolbox. If I unpacked it, people would wander into my room (I had an 'open door' policy at all times so that riders and staff felt they could call on me when they needed) and say, 'It's chaos, Doc!' but everything had its place. If someone well meaning tidied it for me then I wouldn't have a clue where anything was. It was the same with my medical room back at base. Visitors would say that it looked like the room of a disorganised nutty professor, but I knew where everything was.

Anyway. From out of my holdall I'd prepare a daily bag with what I needed for the race, while on the bus I'd have a little store of what I might need afterwards, which would be painkillers, ibuprofen, strappings and tape, antiseptic, dressings, zinc nasal spray, oral zinc, in case they were developing an upper respiratory tract infection, maybe something for the treatment of indigestion, bowel spasm or diarrhoea, spare inhalers and more.

So that was my set-up. As to the task ahead of me? Well, just as I benefitted from Allardyce's more progressive attitude at Bolton, so I did with Brailsford's. He had come into the world of cycling as a new broom, changing the way that riders trained. When he'd first started at British Cycling, a training regime was all about the hours logged. Indeed, there was a story – it might have been apocryphal – of coach Shane Sutton training a group of academy kids in Australia. They were supposed to go out for six hours but it was throwing it down with rain and so they came back after five.

They were just getting off their bikes when Sutton appeared on the front porch of the place they'd rented, yelling at them, 'Go on, you fuckers, get off, you've got another hour to do!'

Brailsford changed all that. He made the training much more specific and scientific: 'You want to win the Tour de France? There's a big mountain, you know how steep it is, let's train on that.'

My background as a GP, training in sports and exercise medicine and my grounding in osteopathy had opened my mind to new ideas in medicine. I wanted to extend ways of thinking I'd begun to explore at Bolton, ways of looking at medicine that differed from the traditional biological model. There's no way that Brailsford would have put up with me if I were a crackpot – he's not a man to suffer fools gladly – but on the other hand he was keen to experiment and innovate, and he challenged me to do the same.

Meanwhile, I was different to the established doctors I encountered at British Cycling and Team Sky. If asked if I wanted to go on such-and-such a tour, I'd shrug and say I'd go where I was needed, while other doctors would be jumping up and down with anticipation; cycling had always struck me as a participation sport rather than a spectator sport. What mainly excited me about my new job was the fact that Team Sky was such a new team, which meant that it was a clean sheet of paper. I had the chance to introduce the principles of sports medicine to a sport that was, if anything, just as backward in that department as football had been.

Even with all the excitement of a new start, I was determined to never lose sight of the fact that when all was said and done, I was still a doctor.

Now, to be a good doctor you don't have to be a *brilliant* doctor. But you do need all the usual qualities you'd expect: training, knowledge, skills, trust and respect. Professor Norman Blacklock, who taught me as a student (who was also the Queen's physician), told me, 'You're only as good as your next patient,' while Professor David Charlesworth, my first boss, told me, 'A good doctor is only as good as the last journal he's read.' Meanwhile, my trainer in general practice, Dr Ted Ainsworth, gave me one of my most important life lessons when he taught me always to be the patient's advocate.

I took all this with me into the demanding area of sports medicine, where I knew from day one that while my patients were riders, with the hopes of the nation resting on their shoulders, they were still my patients, and I was going to have to stand up for them.

Sure enough, over the years I would find myself having to fight for extra recovery time, or for riders to be sent home or withdrawn from competition. I sent Froome home from the 2014 Liège–Bastogne–Liège, and Wiggins home from the 2013 Giro d'Italia – not popular decisions at the time, but fair play, I was always supported by management – and I did it because to be a truly effective doctor in professional sport you have to look after the health of the patient short and long term and have that patient's interest at heart above the interest of the sport or the organisation. At the same time you must be mindful of the demands of the sport, so you understand the particular pressures on that particular athlete as well as their personal goals and, ultimately, their dreams.

That's what it was all about, the very basics of 'performance health management'.

4

Another Day at the Office

An introduction to the physiology and
psychology of the athlete

IF BRAILSFORD WAS TEAM SKY'S inspiring general, and Sutton the gruff sergeant major, then Dr Steve Peters was our cerebral tactician.

Dr Peters, who went on to write *The Chimp Paradox*, a mind-management programme, had spent thirty-five years as Medical Director at the high-security psychiatric hospital Rampton, dealing with mass murderers, rapists, paedophiles, all sorts. So as you might imagine, dealing with athletes as Head of Medicine at Team Sky and British Cycling was a walk in the park after that lot. It was from him that I learned an awful lot about the psychology of the athlete.

He told me that he could always recognise a psychopath – one in ten of us have psychopathic traits, according to him – and that he always knew when someone was lying.

Dr Peters was invaluable in advancing what you might call the psychological management of the team, helping it to function, keeping a lid on the bitching and infighting that occurs in any high-performing organisation. With skills honed at Liverpool FC and in the English national team, he was a superb conduit between the riding staff and management, meaning we never reached that stage common to football where the manager has 'lost' the dressing room. Not all of the riders engaged with him, but some of the most important ones did, and as I had discovered at Bolton, enlisting the support of the leading athletes gives you access to the rest of the team.

For me, psychology in sport can't really be separated from the physical aspect – it's all part and parcel of it. In my experience, most people who make it in sport are already physiologically and psychologically robust. Going back to Gary Speed, he was a shining example of that. There was something special about his physiology. His ligaments, his tendons, his articular cartilage – it was all so good at looking after itself, as though it was more than usually regenerative.

Jason Kenny was another one. Another low-maintenance athlete, Kenny hardly ever picked up injuries and rarely needed treatment – and he's one of the most successful athletes in British Cycling. This, of course, has much to do with Kenny's psychological approach to the sport; he looked after himself. He paid close attention to nutrition and recovery.

Others less genetically blessed were struggling. They were always on the treatment table, always having scans. As a result, they were less successful.

Did Kenny have a better psychological approach because he was physiologically better suited to do so? Maybe. But the fact remains that he knew when he was fit to train.

Another one: Mark Cavendish. I've often attended him when he's crashed at 70km/hour in Lycra. He's never complained about his injuries. Never failed to get back on his bike as quickly as possible. An extremely successful sprinter. Why is that? What makes him so robust and yet so fast? Is there something special about his muscle fibres? I asked him if he'd agree to giving me a muscle biopsy in order that I could put it under a microscope.

'No way, Doc,' was what he said – or words to that effect.

Perfectly understandable, really. A muscle biopsy involves cutting out a piece of muscle. Maybe I'll ask again. I'd love to find out.

Even so, while I'm sure that Cavendish has a unique adaptation of muscle, with presumably a predominance of fast twitch fibres that suit sprinting, I also know that his talent will be multifactorial: physiology, biomechanics, bike-handling, tactics, mental resilience, courage, everything.

I often think about Jason Kenny and Laura Trott in this respect. Great people, great athletes. Both blessed with that combination of physique and psychology that we're talking about. There will be enormous interest in their kids, because we know they've got the genes, it's just a wait-and-see game to discover if they have the attitude too.

It was Allardyce who also taught me a great deal about the psychology of athletes. As I've mentioned, he could take players, primarily with psychological dysfunction rather than physical dysfunction – although the two are connected and one often follows the other – and turn them around. He did it by intuitively knowing when to use the carrot and when to use the stick, when to give a player a roasting and when to support them.

Back to Dr Peters, who could be something of a talisman to the riders, and that was because he exhibited great skill in helping them overcome issues of performance anxiety.

To do this he had a very specific technique, which boiled down to persuading the riders to think of an Olympic final or Tour de France stage as of no more or less importance than a training race – just another day at the office – and approach it in exactly the same frame of mind as a result.

His idea was that we all have several parts to the brain: a human, rational thinking part, an animal emotional (chimp) part and a computer part. The secret was not to let the 'chimp' emotions take over, instead allowing the 'computer' side, where all that training and discipline is kept, to rule. For the riders it was all about discipline and having the belief to trust themselves and their training, almost to stay in rehearsal mode.

I'm at the start line, don't worry about it, I've been at the start line a thousand times.

The start clock is going to bleep. Don't worry about it, the clock has bleeped countless times, I like the sound of the clock.

To underline this philosophy, he told the cautionary tale of a cyclist who, when his rival unexpectedly posted a brilliant time, panicked and changed his gear ratio.

The gearing on a track bike is fixed for the race but can be altered by changing the size of the front chain ring. Sprinters will often look at what gears rivals are using, which is what happened in this example. Our panicking sprinter asked his mechanic for the same gear as his rival. He flunked.

Now, of course, the rider shouldn't have changed his gear ratio. But that was only a symptom of his *real* mistake, which was a failure to believe in himself and trust his training and preparation. Had he done that, he would have won the gold medal.

What Peters instilled in the athletes was a belief in their ability. So much so that riders were coached never to blame themselves, always other outside factors.

The idea being that they would be almost immune to self-doubt, and could then move on quickly after defeat, in order to prepare for the next challenge. Achieve the next goal.

The key – and this is something that we can all benefit from – is to set yourself achievable 'goals' in order to fulfil a bigger 'dream'. But don't concentrate on the dream, concentrate on the goals that build towards it.

That was his model. He promoted it heavily, and his fame soon spread, helped by his television appearance at London 2012. He shared 'the medical apartment' with myself and the physiotherapist and often would be first up heading for the BBC studio. He left cycling in 2012 to go into more mainstream psychology, mostly as a result of his hugely popular book, *The Chimp Paradox*.

His presence was really missed, not just by the riders but by the staff too. A truly remarkable, original mind.

During the time he was my boss he was also my mentor, and from him I learned a lot about how to deal with athletes and coaches. For his part, Dr Peters knew very little of musculoskeletal medicine. Together we were able to look out for all obstructions to an athlete's performance, be they physical or mental.

Any effective athlete is a selfish individual, and riders are no different. They're very self-absorbed, occasionally arrogant and usually obsessed enough to practise what they do for hours on end. They tend to have an innate confidence in their own abilities – although, of course, that could be shaken, which is where Dr Peters came in – and I've met one rider who says they know from the first turn of the crank of the final finishing sprint if they're going to win or not: Mark Cavendish.

But underlying everything – and this applies to Cavendish, Wiggins, Chris Froome and the rest – is the belief that they are the best. Chris Hoy at the 2012 Olympics knew that he was the best in the world; he knew he was going to get a gold medal and in that final race in the keirin he passed through a gap that nobody else could have passed through in order to win the gold medal that capped his career as the most successful Olympic cyclist of all time. And that was all down to belief – belief that was instilled in him – or at least reinforced – by Dr Peters.

Hoy was probably the rider most influenced by Dr Peters, in fact. The other one was Victoria Pendleton.

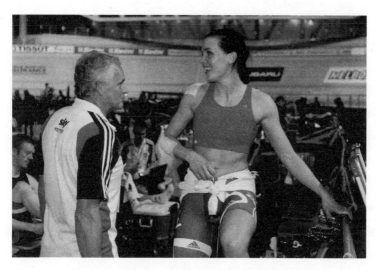

Dr Steve Peters with Victoria Pendleton CBE at the track
world championships, Melbourne 2012.

One thing I had learned as far back as my time at Bolton is that every athlete always has a nemesis, and Pendleton was no different. A very talented rider, she had an almost palpable fear of an Australian sprinter called Anna Meares. But for her biggest competitions, the 2012 World Championships and the 2012 Olympic Games, Dr Peters made her believe that Anna Meares was beatable – if she did her best, and stopped thinking of her.

The other thing to consider if you're interrogating the psyche of the rider is toughness. We tend to think of toughness as a physical attribute, but of course mental toughness is just as important, and you can't have one without the other.

Most of the elite riders I worked with had already been self-selected by their success in amateur sport, by which I mean that they tend to have a very well-functioning body and mind, and are intensely competitive, not just against other people but themselves. That physical and mental toughness was almost always present in the professional athlete, way before they got to me, simply because they needed to have it and had been working so hard at it for years.

Another tried-and-trusted method for increasing mental performance is to rehearse, especially the situations likely to lead to performance-related anxiety. Rehearse and rehearse until it becomes second nature and you believe in your ability to do whatever it is that you're doing, so that you don't *think* but you *know*, that it is reproducible, within your control and if you can do that, you're unbeatable.

A common misconception is to think that you should visualise success in order to achieve success, but this is something in particular that Dr Peters advised against. You should never visualise yourself winning a race. It's the process, achieving the goals set and practised, not the outcome, the dream. Instead what you should visualise is being *prepared* for it; how well you know the start and the thousands of practice starts you'd already done prior to that moment. And everything else – the lure of the top step on the podium, the TV interviews, sponsorship deals, fame, the fortune, the loved ones in the crowd – is put to one side, because you're not at the Olympics, you're at the velodrome doing a practice race with just a man having a cup of coffee sitting in the stands and a cleaner doing the rounds. You're focused; you're doing what you've rehearsed a thousand times, and your heart rate is no higher than it would be in practice. You've got this.

This, of course, feeds into a cyclist's commitment and dedication, the one being the same as the other and both of them always present in the professional cyclist. Geraint Thomas and Peter Kennaugh used to joke about coming back from the January Majorca training camp and having to ride around Manchester in the dark and damp.

'No chance,' they'd say.

But they did.

As I said, just try keeping a rider off his bike.

It was the same with the coaches. Friday afternoon, they'd still be there with their stopwatches, putting on a session, and they'd never cut the session short. Never. The riders wouldn't expect it, probably wouldn't even allow it. Going round again and again.

Not everything always goes to plan, of course; plans can be sent to pieces by certain things, breakages being one of them.

The British Cycling supplier Cervélo had had a problem with their new frame T5GB, pre Rio 2016. The frames weren't strong enough. The sprinters were so powerful, they were breaking their frames in training, while the endurance riders were finding that the handlebar extensions were too fragile to support their arms. Many reverted to training on their old UK Sport Institute (UKSI) funded frames, which were way-ahead-of-their-time black frames made from a carbon fibre and designed in 2002 by the Greek ex-sprinter Dimitri Katsanis, an engineering genius.

It was our mechanics, particularly Ernie Feargrieve, who turned things around. It was like a bike factory at the holding camp at Newport, where the mechanics did amazing work, mending and fettling the bikes in order to make them race-worthy.

Even so, it wasn't enough for some riders, who remained on their trusted UKSI frames for the Games, and this showed the psychological aspects at play. Our mechanics had done great work and the frames were fine from that point onwards. But in the mind of some riders they were 'broken'.

The road riders were what I called the hard men. They'd been through the school of hard knocks, they could live out of a suitcase, and they could look after themselves. But the British Cycling riders were sensitive, maybe partly because they were also younger, but they'd squabble and fall out and take criticism from a coach or a colleague badly.

Dr Peters was good at smoothing over and sorting out that kind of stuff, as was his successor, a psychologist called Dr Anderson who used much more traditional psychological interventions. She was a good listener, full of common sense. She became almost like an agony aunt to a lot of the young female riders, and a very effective member of the team. That's testament to the importance of mental health and psychological support.

Putting together the physiology and psychology, and there's no doubt about it: great athletes are born. It's about athletic prowess, trainability and recoverability, but also something innate.

However, none of that's any good unless there's an amazing will to compete, to train, to win.

The worst part of being at Bolton was the end of every season, when the academy players were released. They'd seen the Premiership footballers, their riches, their fame, only to be told, 'It's not for you.'

I didn't know anything about football. They all seemed so good to me. How could they really tell the difference?

I asked Allardyce about it, and he told me that they were looking for something else, over and above mere skill, some robustness or edge, a desire to work hard, train hard, sacrifice.

That's what makes a good athlete.

Back at Team Sky, and I had the task of getting to grips with the riders in a purely physiological way. And what I quickly discovered was that they are a truly unique breed.

5

In the Purple Zone

Investigating those physiological aspects unique to cyclists

THEY'RE PHYSIOLOGICAL FREAKS, is the answer. The question (or questions) being, what is it that attracts riders to the sport, what keeps them there and what differentiates them from other athletes? And what exactly is the metabolic acidosis that they supposedly thrive upon?

Muscles, when they're exercised, produce lactic acid. So say you're a runner, and you've finished an 800 metre race, your muscles have become very acidotic and painful and the acid is flushed into the bloodstream to be disposed of. That's when you get that lovely grey-white complexion, you feel awful and think you're going to throw up.

The acidosis inhibits the muscle's ability to contract. It is in effect the muscle's way of limiting demands made upon it. You could run further for longer, but only if you ran more slowly; in other words if you didn't ask so much of your muscles, then you wouldn't get that degree of acidosis.

An ability to continue exercising when your muscles become increasingly acidotic is trainable, but it's also a fact that some people – cyclists among them – are just better at dealing with it and are therefore more successful when it comes to performing through the pain of metabolic acidosis, known as 'the purple zone'.

Some riders get a massive surge of lactic acid in their blood-stream after certain intensity and duration of exercise and it leaves them with that awful feeling of nausea, often accompanied with vomiting, which is well recognised in track cycling.

To temporarily rid themselves of the pain, a rider can take bicarbonate, which is an alkaline buffer and can help to limit acidosis. Of course, it has side effects and some riders can't tolerate these, but even so its use is fairly widespread, particularly in time trialling and team pursuit.

We attempted to make its use more scientific by monitoring just how acidotic a rider became in practice, how much bicarbonate they needed, what the potential deleterious effects of repeated use were. It didn't suit everybody. We had to be careful because some would retain fluid as a result of having the bicarbonate at the time-trial stage, then be carrying excess weight for the following day. Others would get abdominal cramps and diarrhoea. In one particular case, a rider took too much and suffered tetany, which is painful involuntary muscle spasms, and needed immediate medical treatment.

Cyclists have that masochistic streak. And the pain of cycling *is* the pain of metabolic acidosis. At first they report pain as being just pain but after that it's purple pain – and it's that purple pain in which the cyclists live, that twilight zone, that separates them from most other athletes and completely from the man in the street, whose muscles would simply stop working. Cyclists can drive their muscles deeper, they can overcome that so-called purple pain. One reason for this is psychological strength. And I think that's what almost selects some of the riders: psychologically not just physiologically they can better tolerate lactic acidosis.

Mind you, they train for it.

A lot of people think that altitude training in preparation for the Tour de France boosts your haemoglobin by stimulating production of more red blood cells. Whether it does or doesn't improve subsequent performance at sea level – I'm not convinced either way – the effect doesn't seem to last very long anyway.

What I do think it achieves is it helps the rider train in metabolic acidosis, increasing the physiological challenge, subsequent muscle adaptation and consequent advantages.

For the same reason I'm sure that a rower could be a good cyclist – Olympic potential, even – simply because they also operate in similar zones.

Many rowers cross over to cycling, often after career-ending lower back problems. Rebecca Romero joined British Cycling from rowing and won gold in Beijing 2008. Equally, maybe you could take a top cyclist and train them in rowing with the same success.

What can we do about it? Well, knowing how the muscles work allows for training which leads to adaptation which leads to improved performance. The coach will train the athlete specifically to achieve this. At Sky we worked with an Australian sports scientist, Tim Kerrison, who had developed an exercise, Sustained Aerobic Performance, aimed at increasing an athlete's tolerance for lactic acidosis. This type of training stimulates the background metabolic rate so more fuel is burned in the following twenty-four hours, which is good for weight control for everyone.

This is where VO2 max comes in. VO2 max is a term loved by number-obsessed cyclists. It's the maximum amount of oxygen your body can effectively extract from the atmosphere and send to your muscles to be used to burn fuel for them to work, and it's expressed as ml/kg/min.

You are born with a VO2 max. Athletes naturally have a high count but training increases it, as does losing weight. A sedentary adult may have a VO2 max of 50 mls/kg/min. A top cyclist might have one of 97.5.

However, the crucial point to take away is that races aren't won just by having the highest VO2 max values but by being able to maintain it for long periods. How do you increase and maintain it? You train. Training improves so many variables that you can stop counting: the blood supply to the muscles, the number and size of the energy generators in the muscles (mitochondria) and the enzymes carrying out the chemical reactions, buffering capacity, and so on.

Something else about pro riders. They all have excellent cardio-vascular systems.

As any amateur cyclist knows, their resting heart rate will decrease the fitter he or she becomes.

I met the retired road racing cyclist Miguel Induráin at the velodrome, where he was visiting his son, also called Miguel, who was training there for a brief period.

As I sit here writing this my resting heart rate is 70 beats per minute, a fit amateur's reading would be around 60 bpm. Big Mig's? 28 bpm.

The heart and lungs are needed to pump oxygen to the exercising muscles. Genetics determine your maximal heart rate and lung capacity, both of which are greater in elite cyclists. Most cyclists will have max heart rates over 200 bpm. Induráin's lung capacity (and lung capacity is one of the biggest indicators of fitness and health) was 7.8 litres; mine is 6 litres. His maximal cardiac output – which is the amount of blood the heart pumps in a minute, and an indicator of the heart's efficiency is 50 litres per minute; mine is 25.

What training can do for us all is to increase the size of the heart's four pumping chambers and make the heart muscle stronger. This effect is then demonstrated by the slowing of your resting heart rate as the pump is more efficient.

All amateurs should determine their maximum heart rate. You will require a heart rate chest monitor. Exercise rapidly, increasing intensity to exhaustion over a few minutes, really to the limit, you must feel like you can't give any more. Then train with a heart-rate monitor.

As you get fitter, your heart rate will not increase to the same extent from the same amount of effort, and it will recover more quickly after exertion. Also record your resting heart rate before getting out of bed in the morning. You will see a gradual reduction in the values, because fitness causes a gradual shift to a slower pulse. However, over-training, under-recovery or possibly an imminent infection will show up as a rising rate. Do you have the start of a sore throat or cold? Well, back off from your training as you'll not benefit from it.

We will return to this in chapter 20, on training schedules.

We always regularly assessed riders' cardiac function with a clinical heart examination, ECGs and echocardiography, and their respiratory functions with spirometry, and they always had what we call athletic hearts, so they are different to the general population.

Then, of course, there's the mind of the cyclist. And again, I come back to this enormous commitment they have. This drive. Riders focus exclusively on cycling and they don't do anything that will affect their recovery, so you won't find them on the golf course after training, they'll be adapting and recovering. One of the endurance girls wouldn't even go shopping when she was training; she'd make her partner go, because she didn't want to stand in the checkout at Tesco.

And if that makes them sound a bit limited, well, nothing could be further from the truth. There were some extraordinarily bright sparks on the team. What they did have was the willingness to be totally selfish, to put their lives on hold. And I loved them for it. There was a purity in what they did because it wasn't done for financial gain. They truly wanted to be the best in the world, they wanted to create a legacy and inspire the nation.

I remember my last Tour of Britain in 2015, which started in my home town of Clitheroe. In 2010, when I started working in cycling, I never could have imagined sitting on a 'Team Wiggo' deckchair drinking coffee on the closed-off High Street. They'd shut the schools, and screaming school kids lined the route; there were Union Jacks everywhere. It was even sunny.

There was a buzz for cycling in Britain and more people had taken it up as a hobby, which of course is great for the nation's overall happiness and health. The riders were all aware of that; they weren't just thinking of racing that day but they were thinking of how they'd changed their nation.

Still, let's not get carried away. Ask the partner of a rider if they're selfish or not. Ask Cath Wiggins, for example. 'Is Bradley a selfish person?'

'No, not when it comes to his wife and family.'

'When it comes to his cycling?'

'Oh, yes. He's a right selfish bastard when it comes to the cycling.'

6

Case Study: Philip Hindes, British track sprint cyclist

Lactic acidosis in action – or was it?

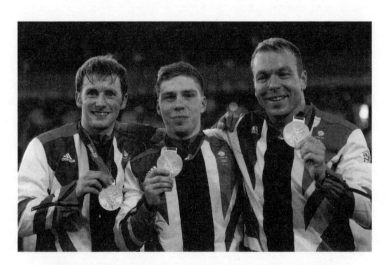

Phillip Hindes MBE, Olympic track team sprint champion
London 2012, Jason Kenny CBE left, Sir Chris Hoy right.

The Line

PHILIP HINDES CAME TO BRITISH CYCLING as a seventeen year old, having obtained British citizenship. He had huge muscles, and he always seemed to be vomiting after intense exercise.

Vomiting. As I said, you see that a lot at cycling competitions. Riders finish and can't even wave to the crowd. They look awful, and the reason is because they're in massive lactic acidosis.

Next thing you know, 'Boke!' and the camera swings politely away. So many times I'd be standing at the end of the race with plastic bags ready to discreetly pass to them. Phillip Hindes would always be like, 'Doc, come here!' and I'd think, *Oh, here we go*. I'd always have a plastic bag on hand for him to puke into.

Now, of course, it's worth reiterating that lactic acidosis is, for most if not all cyclists, a badge of honour, something to be tolerated and dominated.

At British Cycling, it was routine to investigate, and we did a lactic acid profile, took sequential blood samples, several of them in fact, after different types of training.

What transpired was that Hindes wasn't an excessive lactic acid producer – and yet he was feeling excessively unwell with it.

The coaches decided that 'it's because we're training him harder, we're training him deeper at British Cycling, he'll get used to it, he'll adapt'.

But he never did and it became a performance-influencing issue. He was only trained to ride for seventeen seconds per event. His was the starting lap of a three-lap team sprint, so all he had to do was start, finish the first lap and pull off out of the way of man two and that was his race over. But even so, after seventeen seconds he was gone. 'Boke!'

Case Study: Philip Hindes

The problem was that A) it's not very nice to be puking all the time, and B) when you vomit you lose all sorts of essential minerals, particularly potassium, which is a very important electrolyte. We'd try to replace it, but he'd vomit again. We'd try to refuel him, but we found ourselves having to step smartly back after that, too.

I thought, *This isn't lactic acidosis, I don't care what anyone says. This is something gastrointestinal, related to his bowel.*

But what do we do? He had no bowel symptoms any other time.

So I discussed it with a radiologist and we decided to test him in hospital. This had never been done before, in my experience. We arranged for him to bring his bike and turbo trainer into a private hospital and started him exercising – maximal effort, to the point where he knew he would vomit afterwards.

Nausea, some pain, no vomiting. We performed imaging of his stomach immediately afterwards – something called a barium swallow, where he took X-ray contrast material orally, and we used an image-intensifier to follow its progress as it entered the stomach and then went into the small bowel.

At first the fluid passed through him quite normally, until there seemed to be a slight hold-up in the stomach. Oh, that's uncomfortable, pass me the vomit bowl.

He always had a problem if he ever tried to have solid food after a race. Also he had more abdominal pain than was usual with lactic acidosis.

So, we repeated the test again, got him on his turbo, maximal effort, and then we gave him some bread coated in this same contrast material in order to mimic the effects of solid food. He swallowed it and immediately the stomach went into spasm. You could see the stomach filling and a gas bubble forming. *Boke.*

So this lad wasn't suffering from lactic acidosis, he was suffering from a very unusual condition, gastric fundal spasm after exercise.

Next we went down the corridor to speak to another colleague, a very experienced gastric surgeon, Dr Rob Watson, whom I'd known from when I was in general practice. He looked at the images, knew what was happening, and was able to advise us on how to help him. We modified Philip Hinde's hydration and fuelling strategies before training or racing, and used medication to break the vicious cycle.

Once again riders are patients first and athletes second, and I always had to remind myself of that. Sure, they often needed – or just wanted – to train and compete when ill or injured, but it was my job to risk-manage the short-term consequences and think of the longer-term consequences, remembering that they are just human, not super human. I had to try to take a step back from their performance-focused world and stay grounded.

I was probably the only one clocking on at the medal factory permitted to do that.

7

If You Want to Test a Drug . . .

Riders have specific needs when it comes to
vitamins, stimulants, supplements and medicines.
Some are more crucial than others, but they all
require monitoring by yours truly

DURING THE DOPING ERA, riders were incredibly unhealthy; most would take amphetamines (and some worse) and then try to level out with sleeping pills, their one nutrient concession being a vitamin injection. By the time Team Sky started, things were very different, of course.

But I had a lot to learn. For a start, I was shocked at the caffeine use.

Coffee is a substance beloved of cyclists. They love caffeine because it's calorie-free, so they go out for a bike ride, have a nice drink of coffee, get a little bit of mental stimulation without any calorific penalty and then crack on.

Personally, when I go out with my cycling club, I have piece of cake as well as a coffee, but the pros don't, and left to their own devices they'd take on an extraordinary amount of caffeine, whether in coffee, gels, tablets, chewing gum or whatever else is at hand.

The problem is that caffeine isn't great. It's addictive. It causes spikes in heart rate and insulin production. It has been shown to improve psychomotor performance and muscle endurance. I puzzled over why it wasn't banned by WADA. Initially there was a rule that you were only allowed a certain amount in your urine but then that was scrapped and you were allowed as much as you wanted.

My fear of the riders having too much caffeine, aside from its diuretic and dehydrating effects, was because of the risk of cardio-vascular side effects. After all, it is a stimulant, and the riders were consuming it in whatever form they could. So part of my job became to restrict its intake. At Bolton we did it by simply using caffeine-free coffee beans in the canteen grinder, without telling the players, only switching to caffeinated beans on the day of a match.

In cycling it was much more difficult to change what was an incredibly ingrained coffee culture, but gradually as they got to know me and I got to know them, I was able to persuade them of the science behind it, and I managed to get a lot of them to be caffeine free – or at least to have a caffeine washout for a few days before a race or a major event, particularly track events which were usually one-day affairs.

Secondly, there was the amount of supplements riders were taking.

If You Want to Test a Drug . . .

Broadly speaking, I'm against supplements. Yes, some are needed for optimum health (Omega 3, vitamin D and iron for example) but there's no need for all the trace minerals, other vitamins, beta-alanine, creatine, colostrum, branched-chain amino acids, taurine, L-carnitine, and so on.

Part of my job was to (try to) limit their use. I was constantly aware of the WADA code and UK Anti-Doping (UKAD) advice, which is to be wary of contamination. Sport is littered with cases of inadvertent supplement contamination, and the fact is that it's almost always preventable, for the simple reason that most of the supplements themselves are unnecessary. In sports medicine we're all about getting the basics right, and if your diet's good, you don't need this range of supplements.

When I first started, I realised that I was going to have to learn a lot about cycling, because you're only really effective in sports medicine if you understand the needs of the sport and this was all new to me. I saw that this job was about understanding the demands of training and the physiological effects of it, and the use of caffeine and supplements was an intrinsic part of all that because the simple fact of the matter was, the riders loved taking supplements. There was an offensive joke that if you want to test a drug, you give it to a cyclist and supplements were no different. Not funny at the time and it's certainly not funny now.

However, they were legal substances, classified as food supplements. I'd be working on reducing the intake by stealth – exclusion of most supplements was the long-term goal – but in the meantime, my job was to make sure that there was no chance of

69

contamination from wherever they were purchased. So myself and Nigel, the nutritionist for Team Sky and British Cycling, immediately banned the purchase of supplements sourced from the internet, usually from China, and set about confirming a reputable supplier. We used a company which had a monitored supply chain for ingredients and we regularly batch tested their products for contamination. We advised all our riders to use them.

There was one exception. I could always see where this particular rider had been sitting trackside during training or competition, as there would always be a nearly full bottle of protein shake left behind. They'd gulp some down half-heartedly and leave the rest. At the football club we'd provided a pint of milk post match as a protein source.

I told the rider they'd end up at Accrington Stanley. They looked back at me blankly, far too young to remember that old Milk Marketing Board advert (look it up on YouTube).

'How about a pint of milk, post racing?'

'Okay. If it's strawberry flavoured.'

So that was that, a simple marginal gain. I was fine with it. In fact, I'd say to amateur riders, 'Forget spending twenty pounds on a pot of protein powder, you can just have strawberry-flavoured milk.'

The problem is that we've been fooled into thinking that taking supplements is intrinsically sporty. It's part of what I like to think of as the 'medicalisation' of sport, and while it makes money for the supplement company it is not key to athlete welfare, something that runs counter to what I believe in.

* * *

Iron is on my list of approved supplements – for the simple reason that athletes need a lot of it. Why? Well, one of the – forgive the pun – ironies of professional sport is that it's often not at all healthy, and a good example of why this is, is the depleted iron stores of the elite athlete.

Iron is an essential element required for health, and one that is easily obtained through diet. We all know it's required to create haemoglobin in red blood cells in order to carry oxygen in the blood, but it's also needed by muscles in order to produce the energy required for contraction.

A typical body has 3g of iron. Two thirds is found in haemo-globin in the blood and in myoglobin in muscles. One third is in the liver, spleen and bone marrow (where the new red blood cells are made). Lose two litres of blood in an accident (you have just five litres in total, so take care of it) and you will effectively have lost your entire store of iron. By way of comparison menstru-ation loses 30ml – that's approximately 15mg – per day.

Iron is lost in sweat and the destruction of worn-out red blood cells, while for elite endurance athletes the stress of exercise is also responsible for the loss of 3ml of blood per day through bleeding from the gut, and intravascular haemolysis into the urine (haematuria). The levels of the hepcidin, a hormone needed to absorb iron from the gut, also decrease.

All this leads to depletion of iron stores and, eventually, an iron deficiency, also known as anaemia. You can usually tell someone suffering from anaemia: a pallid complexion, breathless-ness and exhaustion are the usual symptoms, as well as a greater susceptibility to minor coughs and common colds.

In athletes it's characterised by loss of performance, which is of course reflected in the numbers that riders love so much: peak and sustained power outputs and split times, heart rates rising faster and higher during exercise with a slower decline after exercise. But crucially it affects the muscles, with difficulty recovering from intense effort, producing muscle fatigue.

Rest reverses the situation and the body restocks itself quickly enough, but if you're a rider in training or racing a Grand Tour, that's not an option. Instead you have to work on increasing intake from the gut, to avoid the loss, which means consciously seeking out food that is rich in iron, particularly if you're a vegetarian or vegan.

An average healthy diet will provide 20mg of iron from which 2mg will be absorbed for the body to use. Red meat and liver are particularly rich, cereals, egg yolk, and green vegetables are useful sources, too. Supplements are of course common in medical practice, particularly iron sulphate in the antenatal clinic. The side effects are nausea and constipation, not good for the elite performer so other products have to be taken to offset these.

I used to provide water naturally rich in iron from a source in the Welsh mountains, which was easy on the gut, but I now use a much more conventional and higher strength formulation, iron bisglycinate, which can be taken in tablet form and is very kind to the gut. Take it at bedtime with vitamin C, which increases the absorption.

Seeing how the athletes relied on all these supplements brought home to me the importance of 'the placebo effect' in this environment.

The placebo effect remains one of the most baffling mysteries in medicine. It was first discovered during drug trials comparing the effects of a real drug against a harmless, useless sugar pill. Half the patients would be given the real drug while the remainder would take the sugar pill, and the effects recorded. The pills would then be switched without the patients' knowledge.

The effects were remarkable, with recipients of the sugar pill – the placebo – not only reporting an improvement – which could simply be a psychological issue – but actually *displaying* a physical improvement.

Meanwhile, a study on a new asthma inhaler in 2011 showed that while the patients' lung function tests did not improve with the placebo non-active inhaler, they reported feeling better. Of course, all asthmatics need inhaled corticosteroids (preventers) and beta agonists (relievers), but it demonstrates the placebo effect.

This placebo effect has been shown to be effective in conventional, complementary and alternative medicine. Though it's unethical to deliberately mislead a patient, the effect can be used to provide care whilst doing no harm nor denying conventional, clinically proven treatments. Riders are particularly susceptible to the placebo effect, as I was to learn – and not just in the realm of food supplements.

In the beginning at Team Sky, riders were permitted to consult their own personal doctor but asked to keep me involved, and later on it was insisted on contractually. They were free to consult their own personal physician, but it had to be with the knowledge of the team doctor, in order to cut down on the risk of them having treatments that might compromise their performance or, worse, inadvertently breach the WADA code.

When it came to self-management of minor ailments though, I insisted on always being involved, and that was simply to eliminate the risk of what we knew as 'the Alain Baxter effect' (we do like an 'effect' in medicine).

The Alain Baxter effect, in a nutshell, is the possibility of athletes accidentally using a banned substance in an over-the-counter medicine. It goes back to the unfortunate case of Scottish skier Alain Baxter, who in 2002 was stripped of his bronze medal when he tested positive for methamphetamine. He was later able prove that the source of the methamphetamine was a Vicks inhaler that he'd bought over the counter while in the United States, having no idea that Vicks in the US differed from the Vicks he had been using at home. Though he remains stripped of his medal he has since launched a campaign to get it back, with thousands of supporters signing an online petition.

The Alain Baxter effect is the reason that any restocking of medicines always comes from the medical facility in Manchester rather than being bought locally at a race.

Need I say that new stock is often delivered in Jiffy bags? Hundreds of them.

The Alain Baxter effect is also the reason that riders are issued with a pack to deal with so-called minor medical problems at home and that includes Strepsils for sore throats, Difflam Oral Rinse, which is an antiseptic painkilling rinse for throat infections, zinc lozenges and nasal sprays, paracetamol, Imodium and cough suppressants, usually Benylin. And again, if these packs needed restocking we'd do so from home so we knew where the contents were sourced from and could be confident that we weren't going to run into any problems with inadvertent breaches of the WADA code.

Although I drew the line and didn't police the content of their wash bags, I was however involved in face care. It's well known that female sprinters can have problems with acne. This is because they do a lot of weight training so that they can effectively be power lifters on bikes, which in turn increases the body's production of testosterone, the muscle-building hormone, and increased levels of testosterone in women commonly causes acne.

So the treatment of acne then became part of my role, just as preferred or optimum menstrual control, saddle-related symptoms and the attempts at the prevention of osteoporosis due to athletic amenorrhoea (which is having no periods due to calorie deficit) all came under my remit.

Some women performed better when they were menstruating, some less well. Sometimes a woman prefers not to be menstruating when she's racing in a Lycra skin suit, for obvious reasons but also for mechanical reasons, in other words the interaction of the saddle and sanitary protection.

People say, 'Doc, you must have been busy with all those illnesses and injuries,' but on the whole they're very healthy people, not permanently ill or injured, so in fact much of my work involved coordinating the whole of the sports science support team: nutrition, physiotherapy, Pilates – all the different inputs. I was effectively the conductor of this orchestra, linking the medical staff with the coaches and Brailsford, and always wary of treading that line between making genuine sporting gains and treating the athletes as normal patients, because that's of course that's what they were to me. Even if I was at the time only dimly aware of their success on the track, I would still be thrilled for them if they did well, but the main attraction of my job was located in their immediate welfare.

This is one of the reasons I have always clung so tightly to the principle of informed consent, which is basically the idea that the patient must be involved in every aspect of the decision-making.

In the old days, Sir Lancelot Spratt would say, 'Your leg's going to have to come off, it's coming off at 9am on Monday,' and tell his staff, 'make sure you get the right leg.'

The joke being that they chopped off the right leg when they should have amputated the left.

Informed consent is saying to the patient, 'Listen, that leg, I don't think I can save it. If we leave it on, you could die of gangrene, if I take it off, you're going to need a prosthetic leg and I agree with you, it's your right leg we're talking about, it's not the left leg, it's the right leg. The risks of the operation are that you could die under anaesthetic, you could get a blood clot, you could get an infection. Do you understand that? What do you want to do?'

I remember an incident prior to an event in the 2012 Olympics, when we were in the Olympic village dining hall. With seating for up to 5,000 it was an impressive place, open twenty-four hours a day, serving food from around the world in order to cater for all tastes – it even had a McDonald's. We tended to sit in little national groups, and were having a pre-race meal – always eaten three hours before competing – when one of our riders jumped up from the dining table and threw up in full view of all present.

I thought, *Crikey, what's going on here?* Was this simply anxiety? Did she have the start of food poisoning? And please, please let this not be the start of an outbreak of the feared norovirus because that spreads like wildfire. (You may recall that at the 2014 Commonwealth Games in Glasgow there was such an outbreak. It is extremely infectious and notoriously difficult to kill with hand washing or hand sanitisers. We delayed our arrival at the Games village because of it.)

Back at our accommodation I walked past the open door of the reserve rider. 'I'm fit, Doc, why take a risk on her?' she implored as I passed. Which might sound rather mercenary but in fact was understandable in the circumstances.

We had to make a decision whether or not to put the sick rider on. It was my opinion after examination that the vomiting was most likely anxiety-related. She had performed well in training, was in form and clearly was the first choice to race.

We did not have the luxury of time, to wait and see. Watchful waiting is a mainstay of management in general practice for early mild non-specific symptoms and is in fact good medical practice. My decision might have been considered bad medicine in general practice, but in performance medicine, with informed consent, the stakes are very different and sometimes you have to train or race when you're injured or ill, or think you might be injured or ill. This is the essence of practising medicine in professional sport, making on-the-spot decisions and it was my job to risk-manage her health with little time for watchful waiting or full investigations to be performed.

I advised her that I considered that there would not be a major effect on performance if she responded to the anti-nausea medication, if she kept her electrolyte replacement drink down and it was safe to race, but in the end the decision was hers to make. There's risk of fainting, even collapsing, falling off at speed, bombing in the event. These are all risks to be considered. Informed consent. She was given all the facts and chose her own path, and I'm happy to say it was the right decision.

So that's informed consent. You discuss the situation with your medical adviser and – uniquely in professional sport with a third party – with your coach.

In the case of a Therapeutic Use Exemption or TUE application, that discussion would also take into account expert independent medical advice.

So, a TUE application. A TUE is one of the ways in which we extend what you might call normal-person healthcare to the elite athlete without the risk of the elite athlete abusing normal-person healthcare and gaining a performance advantage. To get one you must apply to the UCI, the Union Cycliste Internationale, the sport's governing body, and you must meet certain criteria, which are:

4.1 An Athlete may be granted a TUE if (and only if) he/she can show, by a balance of probability, that each of the following conditions is met:

1. *The Prohibited Substance or Prohibited Method in question is needed to treat an acute or chronic medical condition, such that the Athlete would experience a significant impairment to health if the Prohibited Substance or Prohibited Method were to be withheld.*

2. *The Therapeutic Use of the Prohibited Substance or Prohibited Method is highly unlikely to produce any additional enhancement of performance beyond what might be anticipated by a return to the Athlete's normal state of health following the treatment of the acute or chronic medical condition.*

3. *There is no reasonable Therapeutic alternative to the Use of the Prohibited Substance or Prohibited Method.*

4. *The necessity for the Use of the Prohibited Substance or Prohibited Method is not a consequence, wholly or in part, of the prior Use (without a TUE) of a substance or method which was prohibited at the time of such Use.*

All in all, we offered what you might call a complete healthcare service to our riders and not just for their sports-related injuries. This suited some of them, but not all, just as the overall environment of the team was welcomed by some but rubbed others up the wrong way. So, while some riders thrived, not every rider who joined Team Sky enjoyed success with the team.

They had to be willing to buy into that bubble lifestyle. They had to be prepared to have their lives micro-managed. Riders would come in fully expecting to have the coaches rule their training and riding, but even then there would be a period of readjustment as they became accustomed to new ways of training, different to what they were used to in what you might call 'traditional' cycling. After that they'd be surprised to find that the rules extended to nutritional management, hygiene, healthcare and sleep schedules. We believed that what we were doing was holistic and innovative, although some of the teams did think that the Death Star was over the top.

8

Project Ouch

*Though fortunately rare among amateurs, saddle
sores are a common ailment for the professional cyclist.
Here's what we did to fight them, and what we
learned from them*

THE PERINEUM, THAT'S THAT AREA between the genitals and
the anus, is a horrible place to examine on a professional cyclist.
It's full of lumps, bumps and discoloration. There are scars, there's
puckering, fresh chafing, abrasions, bruising, tender nodules, even
open sores and lacerations.

All these are what are colloquially known as saddle sores.

I first became interested in the proactive treatment of saddle
sores in 2013, when I was flown out to Majorca in order to drain
an abscess on Bradley Wiggins, so that he could continue training
and hopefully be healed in time for the Giro d'Italia.

It was not long after that that I began thinking about them

in more depth. Specifically, what we could do to prevent them.

This meant, firstly, identifying exactly what they were. After all, they present a rather mixed bag of symptoms. And secondly, if instead of simply expecting, treating and tolerating them, we could do something to prevent them.

A catalyst for the work came when a particular rider phoned me in desperation, his tour plans in jeopardy. 'I can't train with this saddle sore, Doc, it's killing me.'

A plan formed and I had him flown to Manchester with the intention not just of treating him, but also using him to properly investigate just what these nodules, these so-called saddle sores, really were.

First we performed ultrasound and MR scans on our suffering guinea pig. Next we performed a needle aspiration of the nodule. Nothing grew on culture, so we knew it wasn't infected. The conclusion we drew was that the saddle sore was actually an area of fat necrosis – in other words, dead fat cells – not an infection or abscess as had been previously thought. In other words, it was an inflammation of subcutaneous tissues due to necrosis, caused by pressure and hypoxia in the perineum.

We could now approach the problem and prevention more scientifically. Secondary bacterial infection would always be a risk in this region of the body and in really painful cases local anaesthetic cream would still be an unavoidable necessity.

Other saddle-related symptoms? There's a lot of talk in the media about the onset of numbness in male genitalia because of compressive forces on nerves, which can be an issue but is largely avoidable providing your saddle position is right, and you're using the right saddle type and width. This is something we tackled using bike fits (which we'll come to later).

Neither did I see much prostatitis, which is inflammation of the prostate gland, again something that tends to be reported in male cyclists.

However, moving on from this research we started to think specifically about our female athletes who, according to an audit we carried out, were missing a huge amount of training and even racing as a result of saddle-related symptoms.

Of course, female riders suffer from different problems, specifically unilateral labial swelling or vulval tears, which in the past had been treated with local anaesthetic cream, as well as having the patient sit on bags of slushy ice with their legs up the wall.

I'd asked an Australian team doctor what he did for his female riders in this respect, to which he replied, 'Oh strewth, sport, I don't know, I just give them some cream.' Not an especially satisfactory policy, given that in extreme cases female riders have had to have a procedure called a vulvectomy, where the swollen labia is surgically removed. I was particularly keen to see that none of my riders should ever have to go through that.

So along with Team Sky's head of physiotherapy, Phil Burt, and with input from two colleagues at the English Institute of Sport (EIS), we launched 'Project Ouch', aimed specifically at conducting further investigation into saddle-related symptoms and finding solutions for female cyclists.

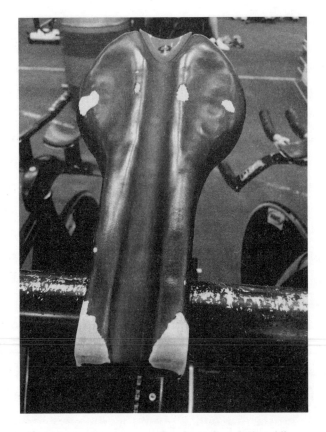

Typical wear patterns on a female track cyclist's saddle.

We sent out questionnaires and conducted interviews, and produced our own research findings. We presented them to an expert think tank, a multidisciplinary team of biological tissue viability experts, gynaecologists, plastic surgeons, tribologists (mechanical engineers expert in friction, lubrication and the wear of interacting surfaces) and dermatologists, even an expert on dealing with boxing injuries to the skin around the eye, not a dissimilar concept concerning the mechanism of trauma.

At the same time, I put a rider who was suffering repeated saddle-related symptoms into an MR scanner with a saddle placed in her riding position, so I was able to see which areas of tissue came into contact with the saddle, an experiment that proved to be extraordinarily helpful.

As a result of all this, we built up a huge research database from which we were able to determine that the saddle-related symptoms that women tended to suffer from, in comparison to the more posterior-placed saddle-sores in men, were labial oedema and labial lacerations, with the latter often coming as a consequence of the former, as a swollen labia is more likely to get caught and torn than a normal-sized labia. These usually needed time off the saddle.

We deduced that the causes were multifactorial: chamois, shorts, saddle, saddle tilt, bike position and personal skin care all played a part, and we were able to pull all the strands together in order to come up with guidelines on the best form of chamois to use, the best form of chamois cream to use, the best soap and moisturiser to use for optimal vulval skin care. The guidelines also included the advice not to shave, but to use a beard trimmer instead, for the simple reason that the presence of some pubic hair will create less friction, while also avoiding microscopic abrasions.

The chamois, incidentally, is the padded insert that goes into the race or training suit. What we realised was that it has to be fitted to the individual. One size does not fit all in this instance – that was apparent from my work in the MR scanner, as well as a pressure-sensitive device that we used on the saddle so that we could tell where each rider was making contact and which areas of tissue were most under stress. From there we worked with the riders to help them choose their own chamois, and made sure that the suit fitted properly at all times, so that even with changes in position – when fatigued or especially when forcibly sitting down after the start – it remained in the optimal position. Kinking and creasing of the chamois especially were involved in labial tears.

It was a labour-intensive, not to mention expensive, period. But fruitful. We employed a designer to make bespoke skin suits for the whole female podium squad, and I'm not exaggerating, we virtually eliminated saddle-related symptoms in women.

Another useful outcome was that we learned that riding with a wet chamois massively increased skin friction and led especially to labial abrasions. We encouraged riders to avoid training in soaking conditions, or change skin suits at a food stop, and to deal with inevitable in-race calls of nature appropriately. For a chamois cream we recommended Epaderm Ointment, and for washing, Dermol 500. The consultant dermatologist, Dr Jane Sterling, produced a very helpful guide to maintaining the skin health of this area and it's in the appendix for reference, should you wish to read more.

As for the amateur, there's much to learn from our findings. We're all different, so the advice is to experiment with trial and error. You will find a position where that saddle interaction with your perineum suits you, and remember that one saddle doesn't suit all – so try before you buy. There are different saddles designed for men and women so get the right one, and always angle it down slightly.

Read up about how to look after your perineum with regard to hygiene, moisturising and recovery. We've talked about recovery, and that part of the body is no different to other areas of the body. Mostly it's so important that if you're doing a lot of road riding, whether you're a man or a woman, that your kit fits properly, that the chamois you choose is comfortable and suits you and the placement is right. Remember that it's supposed to help with the friction against the saddle. Try not to ride with a wet chamois and make sure it always stays in position, doesn't ruck up, doesn't fold, doesn't crease.

The main takeaway is: if you're getting symptoms down below, don't ignore them. Consult your GP, and though they may not have the expertise, he or she can direct you to expert doctors who can give an opinion.

9

Look After Yourself – Sport Isn't Always Healthy

A look at those injuries and complaints common to
all cyclists – and some tips on avoiding them

WHEN I FIRST BEGAN AT TEAM SKY, fresh from football, with absolutely no idea of the issues unique to cyclists, the riders used to take the mick: 'Doc, what have you got for sore legs?' they'd say.

I'd be scratching my head, wondering what I could do for them. More to the point, *Why did they always laugh when they asked me what I had for sore legs?*

The point was, of course, that they all had sore legs all of the time. It's for this reason that legs are afforded the lion's share of the soft-tissue massage, something that takes place on a daily basis.

Muscles love soft-tissue therapy. And because muscles love

soft-tissue therapy the riders like it too, although there's probably a bit more to it than that. All we do know is that it's a very pleasing experience for many reasons that we don't understand but are probably something to do with the endorphins and enkephalins released during the process, which makes the recipient feel better – something we can all relate to from our visits to the spa.

Another massive benefit of the soft-tissue massage ritual was due to the masseurs themselves. It was an opportunity for one-on-one time to chat with a confidant, and was a vital step in recovery.

This led to a very strong bond. Txema González was Wiggins's swanny in 2010. Mark Cavendish used a very interesting man called Aldis, who was in fact a doctor from Lithuania but couldn't get recognition for his medical degree in the EU. His skill set included massage, manipulation, muscle balance techniques and much more, and he travelled from team to team with Cav.

Massage can almost get addictive for the riders, and at British Cycling, where the resources were always more limited, we had to control its use. Unless it was the Olympics, or the build-up to the Olympics, I would have to restrict even the so-called podium athletes, the Chris Hoys and the Victoria Pendletons, to a maximum of two sessions a week. Our limited resources meant that some academy riders would simply have to do without.

Still, a soft-tissue massage would do a lot to relieve those sore legs the riders used to rib me about, which was the point, after all. They have to look after the important muscles – in other words, the muscles at the front of the thigh (the quads), the buttock muscles (the gluteals), and the calves, which are very important in cycling.

Look After Yourself – Sport Isn't Always Healthy

Less important, but not to be neglected, are the reciprocal muscles, the hamstrings and the hip flexor psoas. In track sprinting, the psoas is a more important muscle group. It's important to massage and stretch it after a long bike ride as it tends to shortens and tighten. If you're an amateur cyclist, you should definitely get into the habit of doing that. Some stretches are done lying down, others in a lunge motion. It's probably a good idea to investigate via YouTube or similar as to which stretch is best for you.

Other problem areas? Because of the extreme positions, the lower back would often suffer. Remember, these aren't recreational riders we're talking about here. They race in postures aimed at achieving the optimum aerodynamic profile, which in turn place the lumbar spine under an awful lot of stress.

Now, if they also need to see where they're going, which is advantageous for a cyclist, they have to look up, which means that the cervical spine is in the unfortunate position of being hyper-extended for much of the time. It's a sad fact of life for the two-wheeled athlete that the aerodynamic position is a very uncomfortable and potentially damaging position.

I'd go further and say that one of the reasons that Wiggins has been so successful is that he can preserve an extreme aerodynamic position and still maintain optimal power production from his legs, and that's largely down to the fact that he has very flexible hamstrings which allow him to keep the knee extended and to rotate his pelvis forward to go low at the front. Combined with his narrow shoulders this presents less aerodynamic drag. Most importantly he could maintain this optimal position even when fatigued, something many riders couldn't achieve even with training, stretching and sessions in the wind tunnel.

I should mention, by the way, that power outputs are some of the most closely protected secrets in cycling, the numbers only very rarely released. Wiggins has allowed me to print his power output record (we'll come to this later) from his last race for Team Sky, the 2015 Paris–Roubaix, a 257km day race aptly named 'The Hell of the North' because of its twenty-nine cobbled sections. The power is measured through mechanical sensors in the crank that allow us to monitor output in both legs, the pedal rotation speed (the cadence), and the heart rate through a chest monitor. At the end of the day, the data log from each rider's bike computer is uploaded so that the coach and I can see what stress each rider's been under, how much power he's had to produce for how long and what his heart rate has been.

From that we work out a stress score, add it to what the rider tells us – 'I had a good day,' or, 'I was completely rinsed' – and we could tell how they were going to feel the next day, which in turn affects the coach's tactics.

Returning to the lower back for a moment, and what we found was that sprinters in particular struggled with slipped discs (lumbar disc prolapses) and that was due to loading in their strength and conditioning programmes.

And yes, you did read that correctly. An injury audit by Phil Burt confirmed it: the biggest cause of injury in track cyclists was not out on the track. It wasn't through riding, falling off, or repetitive over-use injuries, it was in the gym, lifting weights.

This was because as a rule, the track cyclists would spend as much time in the gymnasium as on the track. They were effectively strength-and-conditioning athletes, and called 'power lifters on bikes' by some sarcastic endurance riders.

A good example was Chris Hoy, whose lifting and pressing personal bests were phenomenal. He is a perfect illustration of what twenty years in the gym – with no anabolic steroids – can do for you.

When I was in general practice, I'd have patients who, once they realised that my speciality was sport, would confess that they were doping with anabolic steroids and ask for help, not just for side effects but for performance.

Sadly, steroid use is not at all uncommon in recreational gym use, where body builders are attempting to get what they think of as a 'ripped' look, despite the fact that it creates a very characteristic and glaringly obvious pattern of muscle development, and there is excess hypertrophy – i.e. enlargement – over power (or performance) gains.

Not Sir Chris. He's carved out of Scottish granite. The only member of the staff capable of giving his enormous quads an effective soft-tissue massage was the physio Phil Burt, himself a big bear of a man, with appropriately sized hands. Hence he travelled wherever Hoy was competing.

So, yes – the most common injury was lumbar spine problems and that was either prolapsed discs or spinal facet joint inflammation.

A very effective treatment for facet joints involved the CT scanner – computerised tomography – which allowed us to perform an X-ray-generated bone scan, followed by a CT-guided injection of triamcinolone, either directly into the facet joints or into the epidural space around the inflamed nerve root.

These injections were remarkably well targeted; you could see exactly where the needle was going under the computerised tomography guidance. At £1,500, it was costly, but it revolutionised my management of these spinal problems.

As a result of recurring back problems, some athletes couldn't squat in the gym and so had to be protected when they were squatting. We were very innovative in allowing athletes to train the muscle groups the sprint coaches wanted whilst protecting the lumbar spine. One way to do this was using the sitting leg press, single or double, and another way was the track bar dead lift.

When they were rehabilitating from an injury, we used a novel form of training called 'blood flow restricted resistance exercise'. This involved them exercising the muscle group being trained in a physiologically hostile environment to force adaptation, but not with the usual massive loads, hence protection from injury. This was done by producing arterial hypoxia in the muscle group, which in layman's terms means acidosis. So they'd have a band, a bit like a blood pressure cuff, wrapped around the leg or the arm and inflated to above systolic arterial pressure, effectively stopping the supply of oxygenated blood to the muscle.

The results were remarkable. But it was very painful. You try exercising when you have a compressive cuff around your legs. I tried it, found it very uncomfortable and had to terminate my exercise.

Could all the riders do it? 'Sure,' they say, 'Bring it on.'

10

Case Study: Ed Clancy, track cyclist, twenty-two weeks pre-Rio 2016

A lumbar disc prolapse can affect anybody, although it's an injury prevalent in cycling. Trust me, you'll be sitting back in your seat after reading this . . .

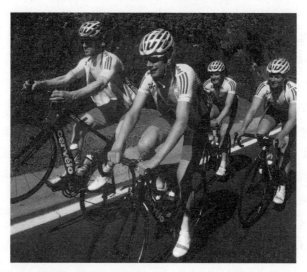

Ed Clancy OBE pulling a wheelie on a recovery ride on Mount Teide, Tenerife 2015, with Andy Tennant, Steven Burke MBE and Jon Dibben.

The Line

THIS WAS A REAL RACE AGAINST TIME.

Ed Clancy made a huge contribution to the team pursuit and indeed is the reigning Olympic, world and European champion in that discipline.

Now, any movement, not just exercise, can put a strain on your lumbar spine and that's why you can be lifting up a chair at home or putting your briefcase in the car boot and suffer acute lower back pain. But for a track cyclist like Clancy the risk of serious damage is increased hugely – there are *massive* stresses on the lumbar spine, particularly at the starts, when riders are turning a big gear from a standing start, generating enormous forces that begin at the handlebars, travel the entire body and combine with the legs in order to produce the power they need at the pedals.

That being the case you'd think that any lumbar injury suffered by Clancy would occur on the track. But in fact he was simply picking up his suitcase after finishing the Tour of Britain when he felt something 'go' in his lower back.

It was as innocuous as that.

The next morning he couldn't move and was suffering pain along his leg. He gave me a call. 'Ah, Doc, its not good, something's gone . . .'

Right away, I'm thinking, *Lumbar disc prolapse.*

Exactly what is that? Well, I always imagine the disks of the spine as the custard in a vanilla slice. If you squeeze a vanilla slice, the custard pops out and that's what happens with a disc. The shock-absorbing material in the disc is pushed out and presses on the sensitive spinal cord or more likely the existing spinal nerve roots – a prolapsed disc.

Case Study: Ed Clancy

It can happen in any number of ways. Plenty of daily activities produce this stress on the lumbar spin. Even just sitting forward eating your dinner, looking at your computer or driving means you're constantly squashing your discs. In short, any excess force in a flexed position – made worse if you add in any rotation of the spine at the same time – and you risk a prolapse.

In the case of Clancy, I started with ice and painkillers, examining him for signs of nerve root irritation or sciatica, which is leg pain from the pressure on the spinal nerves, thinking to myself, *Lets hope this isn't going to need a surgical decompression.*

What's that? Well, in an emergency situation the disc prolapse actually presses on the nerve roots in the lower part of the spinal column that control bladder and bowel function. The patient, forget whether they're an athlete or a member of the general public, will then suffer, not only severe lower back pain, but also dribbling urine incontinence or even faecal incontinence, combined with an absence of sensation around that part of the body, the perineum.

That is a surgical emergency – you've got twenty-four hours to get them to a hospital, see a neurosurgeon, and get that disc decompressed, because if the nerve roots are damaged for more than twenty-four hours, function won't come back and you'd be permanently incontinent.

This dire outcome wasn't the case with Clancy, thank goodness, though he was of course very distressed and concerned about his training plans going out of the window, not to mention being in severe pain.

Needless to say, as a hard-man cyclist he played down this latter aspect. His primary focus was Rio.

The Line

'When can I get back to training?' was his only question. As we'll see, time and time again, my job entailed a delicate balancing act between getting the patient fully recovered and doing it with the minimum disruption to their training. They all want you to be able to wave a magic wand. Clancy was no different.

So I went through the standard procedure. Confirming the diagnosis with an MR scan of his lumbar spine, discussing the case with the radiologist, establishing that it was indeed a lumbar disc prolapse but clinically and radiologically not giving significant compression on the nerve root.

So we're eleven months away from the Olympics, and now we're in a holding pattern, deciding to manage it conservatively and trying to keep a lid on Clancy's expectations.

Firstly, in order to decrease the pain and inflammation we carried out a CT-guided epidural injection of the anti-inflammatory triamcinolone.

Secondly, we kept him moving. For most back problems that's the key. At the same time, his strength and conditioning programme was modified to protect the lumbar spine, and he was soon reintroduced to his bike. He'd be managed by the medical team until he was fit to be thrown back in.

We couldn't solve the disc prolapse itself; that would have to resolve itself naturally. The body has a systematic process of four overlapping phases in healing: haemostasis in a few hours, inflammation over several days, proliferation of new tissue for two to three weeks and then maturation, strengthening and remodelling.

The end point of the final stage is harder to predict, but even when healing is over, the resulting scar tissue is only 80% of its previous tensile strength. So it's never invisible mending.

There will always be weakness. The best predictor of having another lumbar disc prolapse is having had one previously. So sports doctors will do anything they can to enable the body to achieve its own optimum healing potential, and this was one of those occasions where we were simply trying to give the body a helping hand by relieving the pain to allow movement, unloading disc pressure by resting him in certain postures, encouraging blood flow to the spine, maintaining the strength of the core muscles and waiting for the disc extrusion to be reabsorbed. At the same time, we kept his cardiovascular system, his cycling muscles, and his mind from deconditioning too much. Very important, that. If you shut everything down, within three weeks all those gains you've made will start to be lost. Those muscles will atrophy.

As his training stress was ramped up, Clancy's lumbar spine continued to grumble. Clearly there was a persistent problem, and he was worried that he might have to miss the Olympics – as were the coach and squad.

Me? Certainly the Olympics were his dream, the aim of his goals, but it was still sport. I was worried that he might end up with permanent, life-changing damage to his spine.

With twenty-two weeks until Clancy was expected to compete in the qualification rounds for Rio 2016, we consulted an eminent neurosurgeon, Mr Gerry Towns, who routinely deals with lumbar disc prolapse but who had specific expertise in dealing with the extra demands and requirements of elite athletes.

We were in his office as Mr Towns reviewed the scans and talked over the various medical interventions so far. He wanted some time to think. It was a timescale he'd not been challenged by before. And so a short while later I found myself back in his office, discussing surgery.

'I think we should go in,' he told me.

I sat down later with the rider and his coach to discuss all the options and consequences.

In fact, it's a fairly routine procedure. Best done by neurosurgeons, it's called a microdiscectomy: 'micro', as in microscopic; 'disc', that's the lumbar disc; 'ectomy' means cutting out. It can be done with a scalpel but it's usually done with a thermocoagulation laser, which effectively clots, cuts and vaporises tissue and it usually has a good outcome.

On the other hand, it's still surgery; it's still invasive. You don't want to have surgery if you don't have to. There are risks associated with anaesthesia; there's the danger of post-op infection. Plus, you need a period of recovery. You don't have lumbar disc surgery and go straight back to work. You certainly don't go straight back to work if your job is being an elite athlete. Not only that, but the location in the body is what surgeons describe as tiger country – in other words, a very scary place to be – because you've got a spinal column and spinal nerves down there, and if it goes wrong, you risk paralysing the patient.

Mr Towns knew that the timescales were going to be tight; that it was a potential risk.

And so, as ever, it came down to informed consent. I returned with the patient so that Mr Towns could run through the potential benefits and the possible risks of the operation with him. He laid the options on the table. The patient has ultimate control of his body, not the coach, not the team.

There was, as is usually the case, consensus from all concerned: Clancy, his coach, me and the surgeon. We knew that if he didn't have the microdiscectomy, he wasn't going to Rio and even if he had the microdiscectomy, he might not recover sufficiently and be able to continue the training required to go to Rio.

And that was where the risk lay, because Mr Towns couldn't guarantee that if he operated on Clancy immediately he would be fit and ready in time to be on the start line at the Olympics.

And as I said at the time and have said countless times over the years, medicine can't get too clever. You can't cheat the process of physiology, no matter what the rider, coaches or competition demand.

But what you can do – and in the case of an athlete on whom the country has pinned its hopes for Rio 2016, what you *have* to do – is manage it, avoid complications, and at the same time keep all the other functions of the body going as described above.

So it's basically a race against time.

The surgery went ahead with no complications, which was encouraging and allowed us to embark on a managed rehabilitation plan, the goal being to get him to the Games fitter and stronger than ever before, and capable of breaking the world record.

Rehabilitation's hard and it's lonely for athletes because they don't train with the squad; the athlete (as well as the support team) must take ownership, responsibility, be disciplined and committed to the plan. Clancy clearly was, he did everything that was asked of him. Yes, there were little setbacks along the way. Sometimes we perhaps pushed a little bit too fast, a little bit too hard and got some knock-backs, some increasing pain, some sensory disturbance. But he got on track and there's a lovely picture of him taken in the athletes' village at Rio, with his gold medal around his neck and the three people who helped him: Phil Burt, his soft-tissue therapist Hannah Crawley, and me.

All in all, a superb example of sports medicine at work.

11

Case Study: Athlete A

Some tough decisions to be made as a spinal injury puts an athlete at risk of missing the Olympics

AS WE'VE ALREADY SAID, SPRINTERS spend a lot of time in the gymnasium – often it seems more time in the gymnasium than they do on the track.

With road racers, it's all about being out on the road; working on their miles and sustained power outputs. For sprinters, however, it's more a case of keeping several training balls in the air at the same time, which means constantly having to ask themselves whether or not to stay in the gym or get out on the track. Riders in the gym are always having to push, push, push, to force muscle groups into adaptation; in other words a change in the size, structure and function of the muscle groups in order to produce more power for longer.

Squatting weights is the sprinters' exercise of choice to build their gluteals and the quadriceps, and they can and will do it until the cows come home. For the amateur, you can build both just with normal squats, arms outstretched, building up to barbell squats and deadlifts if you're feeling brave. There are also certain lunges that will help.

Leading up to a big event there are some who will taper and finish their strength and conditioning in the gymnasium sooner than others. Most sprinters feel that if they stop too early, they'll lose power for the event. On the other hand, the desired result of adaptation needs time to take effect and the rider needs to recover from the fatigue it generates.

The real problem with strength-and-conditioning training is that it tends to be when the majority of injuries occur. It's a risky endeavour as we've discussed, particularly squatting as they would lift phenomenal amounts. Liam Phillips the ex-BMX world champion would squat 215kg whilst weighing 84kg.

Of course, sprint coaches love strength and conditioning for the simple reason that power equals winning in sprint cycling. So riders were constantly at the limit, and it was always a case of calculating how much stress they could put through the spine and the power producers: the glutes and quads.

To protect the lower back from damage sustained during weight training, Phil Burt, and our strength-and-conditioning coach, Martin Evans, put a lot of work into constructing exercise programmes that could produce the adaptations and strength gains required for success on the track while ensuring they got to the start line. They invested heavily in equipment for the gym for their innovative approach to be successful, particularly the single and double leg press.

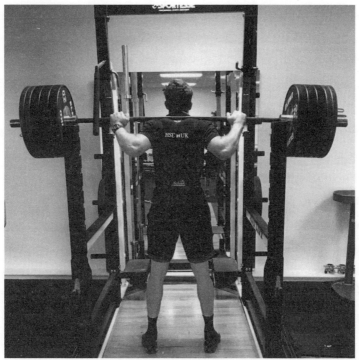

Liam Phillips, BMX world champion, squatting in the gym at the
Manchester velodrome.

Meanwhile, the medical team would be constantly monitoring riders in the gym, ensuring an appropriate warm-up,
and we'd intervene early if there were any concerns. Obviously
if riders showed poor technique or experienced any symptoms,
then that was an alert and could shut down the session.
Ultimately, Hannah Crawley the soft-tissue rehabilitation therapist would attend each session in the gym to also constantly
monitor the riders.

So, that's how we managed them in the gymnasium, and for
this reason it was important that the strength-and-conditioning
team liaised effectively with the medical team, in order to produce

maximum strength gain with minimum musculoskeletal injury. A frequent injury was facet joint inflammation.

Which is? I'll explain. The spine has thirty-two vertebrae and each vertebra has two facet joints, an upper and a lower on each side, at the back of it, which direct the movement of the spine, with each facet joint connected to the facet joint above and below. In weightlifting it becomes a weight-bearing joint, which is not what nature intended, and puts it at great risk.

And so we come on to Athlete A.

Four weeks before the Olympics, Athlete A's lower lumbar spinal facet joints were very inflamed, and it was so bad that I was thinking they certainly wouldn't be able to continue training at the required level and even getting to the starting line at the Games was in jeopardy.

'Doc, I've got too much back pain,' the rider reported. They were matter-of-fact about it but the pale, tense face told its own story.

Some athletes know their body so well that they know if something serious is wrong.

Professional sport hurts. Every training session hurts. Sure some are oversensitive, some fondly known as hypochondriacs, some need to complain and have continuous reassurance. These often required a 'reassureagram', a harmless, but expensive, MR scan for a symptom which I almost always thought would not reveal significant tissue damage, but was an effective and often necessary management tool. It gives the athlete reassurance to crack on, confident that the pain isn't causing them damage.

Athletes are like racehorses. They're high-performing, high-maintenance thoroughbreds and they need to exercise daily, which means they often have to train or race with injuries of one sort or another.

But unlike animals, riders can talk and tell me their symptoms, and I'm a good listener. Certain symptoms are more worrying than others and paraspinal lower back pain, particularly when it's come on after a gym session, is a big red flag to any medical professional. Even though the examination, apart from some back muscle spasm, was entirely normal.

I didn't mess about. I organised an immediate MR scan at the Ally Pally, the local private Alexandra Hospital, who still gave us fast-track access from my days at Bolton. At the time they would reserve a daily slot for us after training so we didn't have to worry about being fitted in. Equally, they'd be happy to stay late or open up early for us. This being the run-up to the Olympics they were even more accommodating, thank goodness.

Usually the results were sent to my radiologist colleague Dr O'Connor and he'd look at them, either in his office at Chapel Allerton Hospital in Leeds, or at his kitchen table at home, before we'd compare notes. Sometimes, if it warranted it, I'd get in the car and drive to him in order that we could look at the images together, a proper old-style clinical case conference.

On occasions, if we had a particularly complicated lumbar back issue that wasn't settling and were considering surgery, we'd go to a multidisciplinary spinal meeting at Leeds General Infirmary, where experts in pathology, neurosurgery, orthopaedic surgery and radiology from across the whole of the Leeds teaching hospital network would meet on a weekly basis to discuss complex cases.

Athlete A wasn't one of those cases. It was a common problem, inflammation of the facet joints – in this case, one on each side between L5 and S1 vertebrae was inflamed, a significant pain generator and inhibitor of lumbar spine and core stability muscle function – but it needed to be managed effectively and quickly.

Treatment options were discussed and a treatment plan agreed, involving the coach, informed consent from the rider, and keeping the strength-and-conditioning coach in the loop. The goal was simply getting to the start line in London and being as fast as the rider had ever been. We decided to inject the facet joints with the anti-inflammatory triamcinolone. It didn't require a TUE because it was outside competition, specifically more than eight days before the competition was due to start.

So we booked into a private hospital in Leeds the next day, and Dr O'Connor used CT scanning to determine the exact location of the inflamed facet joints (also in tiger country – millimetres from the spinal nerves) and guide the injection directly into them. A radio-opaque dye was included in the injection, so that when a CT scan was taken afterwards, we could confirm the exact, correct location of the drug,

Compare this approach to the one we would have taken in general practice, when you couldn't fast-track it; you wouldn't do an immediate MR scan to confirm an inflamed facet joint and you certainly wouldn't reach for a CT-guided injection of the facet joint as a treatment option.

There'd be a period of relative rest for the patient; there'd be oral painkillers first, maybe some oral anti-inflammatory tablets later and then progression into a physiotherapy-led managed rehabilitation programme. And in the majority of cases, with time and when you removed what caused it – such as lifting heavy weights in the gym – it would settle.

And let's be clear. That would be my preferred course of treatment, because in my opinion that's the *appropriate* course of action. Personally, if I had an acute facet joint injury like that, I'd wait; I wouldn't want a spinal injection for the simple reason that it's an invasive procedure and there are risks associated with it. The needle might not be able to enter the facet joint. There could be haemorrhage. There could be infection introduced into the spinal cord, even meningitis. Then there are the potential side effects of triamcinolone itself, rare though they are. All must be considered.

Again, this is where informed consent comes into it. Athlete A was expected to do very well at the Olympics and had trained very hard towards that one big event. They were at real risk of not competing.

Of course, the rider wanted immediate resolution. In all branches of medicine, when patients are ill, they're either frightened, in pain, have loss of function, or some combination of all three. They're desperate. So a part of my role as a doctor and someone who always strives for good medical practice is to protect patients from unnecessary procedures. Never winning at all costs – yet another of my treasured mantras.

In this case, we all agreed the risk management, and went

ahead with the injection procedure, and we were able to decrease the pain and inflammation and begin a course of effective rehabilitation in conjunction with the sprint coach and get the athlete to the holding camp in top shape. Form was good, too.

And that rider went on to do pretty well at the Olympics.

12

Case Study: Jess Varnish, track sprinter, World Class Performance Programme

Informed consent in action as Jess Varnish considers the risks involved in her treatment . . .

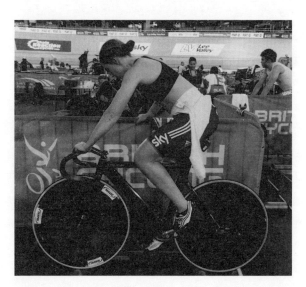

Jess Varnish track sprinter warming up on rollers, Lee Valley velodrome.

The Line

VARNISH HAD A LUMBAR SPINE PROBLEM, but it wasn't managed surgically. Again, it was the usual thing: while in the gymnasium, she developed pain in her lumbar spine that prevented her from continuing – at which point she became our responsibility.

I performed an MR scan, which confirmed a disc prolapse. Now, this wasn't an Olympic year – it was 2013 – but her goal was to perform at the World Championships that year. Her goal was a further step to her dream: winning Olympic gold.

'I need to go, Doc,' she told me. 'They'll cut my funding if I don't hit my target performance at the World Championships.'

There are always other agendas.

I said, 'Well, listen, there are . . . *issues* involved with having a CT-guided epidural injection. On the one hand, the risks decrease with the experience of the person doing it and the use of the gold-standard imaging and image-guided injection. You can't get better than CT-guided injection for epidurals with an experienced interventional musculoskeletal radiologist – and you'll be getting the best. So the risks are minimised.'

'But there are risks?'

'You have to be aware of them. There could be haemorrhage. There could be infection. There could be paralysis.'

That gave her pause for thought.

As I say, had it been an Olympics year, I think it would have been a very different scenario. Almost certainly she would have insisted on having a CT-guided lumbar epidural, the coaches and management would have pushed for it as well. But it wasn't the Olympics, just the World Championships, and it was my opinion that it wasn't worth the risk.

'It isn't a surgical emergency and it has not yet become a chronic problem,' I told her. 'This is a first occurrence that treated properly will heal itself pretty damn well. It needs time.'

She could have pushed it had she'd wanted to. If she'd done that, then maybe myself or the musculoskeletal radiologist would have told her, 'Okay, forget your sport, I'm going to treat you just as a normal patient now. You have an uncomplicated lumbar disc prolapse, but I advise conservative management, giving it some time for the expected spontaneous recovery. Disagree? Let's arrange a second opinion with another independent expert.' A good doctor, confident in his practice, always encourages the patient to exercise the right to a second opinion.

Ultimately she saw it our way. Athletes, particularly bike riders, are generally sensible people and their bodies are important to them. Yes, there was the blow that she had her funding cut, but she made the right decision, and ultimately she was able to come back, train and compete. In other words, she lived to fight another day.

A good day at the office. Sports medicine working the way it should.

13

And Breathe . . .

Cyclists are more than usually susceptible to respiratory issues. Here we ask: what are those issues, and why do they affect riders in particular?

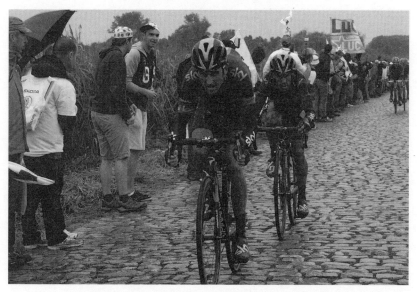

Geraint Thomas MBE with Ritchie Porte over the
cobbles of Paris–Roubaix, 'the hell of the north'.

THE ROAD RIDER'S POST-RACE COUGH was a new one to me – yet another of those conditions that only cyclists seem to suffer.

I'd heard of the Khumbu Cough, which is named after the valley that leads up to Mount Everest and is brought on by the cold, dry air at high altitude. But not the rider's cough, which also seemed to be brought on by a specific set of circumstances: the coldness and dryness of high altitude during a Grand Tour. Pollen from the sunflowers. Muck from the road. The entire road team would be hacking.

So, I thought, what should I do? I did a bit of research and consulted a professor of respiratory medicine. His lifelong interest was the cough and he was working with a pharmaceutical company to manufacture an effective medicine.

His scientific knowledge and passion were obvious as soon as he spoke. He told me, 'If you want some good advice, this cough medicine will be based on menthol. And if you want a good cough suppressant with menthol in now, buy some Fisherman's Friends.' (A good example of KISS, a mnemonic for 'keep it simple stupid' that I often used in medical practice.)

So I took him at his word, bought Fishermen's Friends and it revolutionised our treatment of the rider's cough, so that ultimately a packet of Fisherman's Friends became standard issue to riders when they were training or competing.

The professor went into great detail about the different cough receptors and what stimulates them, but I was just looking to manage the cough, I didn't need to fully understand it.

That was part of my job, to consult with the specialists. I was aware that I wasn't going to be an expert in everything, but I knew who to approach for what.

A similar thing happened when I went to another respiratory physician for advice on the management of airway sensitivity and susceptibility to upper respiratory tract infections. He worked in a heart/lung transplant centre but had published a paper on airway sensitivity and its innovative management that I liked.

He introduced me to the concept of how, why and what happens when the mucosa in the lining of the lung dries out. He described it ultimately as cracking, which was a helpful way of visualising the process, in particular the mucosa's vulnerability to infection, as well as providing the answer as to why one particular rider always seemed to come down with an upper respiratory tract infection when racing in the high, dry mountains.

The specialist was able to offer a treatment for it, which was inhalation of a nebulised solution of hypertonic saline solution – effectively salt in water but more concentrated than exists in the body's tissues, and nebulised means that it is produced as a fine spray.

Whilst it wasn't necessarily a medicine, it was a pharmaceutical-grade product manufactured to a prescribed standard and we did try that with some success with this particular rider. Ultimately, which is often the case, we discovered another more effective management strategy.

Which brings me on to Fluimucil, a medication, also known as a mucolytic, that is designed to break up accumulated mucus. It came to be used for the same reason as Fisherman's Friends – because of a cough.

Rain was always an issue on the tours. On the Tour de France, they sweep the roads each night in order to try and clear the route of debris, but invariably some farmer will send his cattle across the road in the early hours, leaving dung all over the road. Not even the Tour de France can stop the age-old practices of farming.

And as long as the weather wasn't too bad then the riders didn't suffer. The problems arose when the dung got wet. With 198 bikes racing through it, it liquefied and created an aerosol-like effect.

When the riders finished the stage, their faces were covered in muck apart from where they'd been wearing their sunglasses. They looked like old-time racing car drivers. So you can imagine what they'd been breathing in all day: not only fumes from the cars all around, pollen from the fields, but whatever else had found its way on to the road.

Remember, they would have been breathing maybe thirty to forty breaths a minute for six hours through all that.

As a result, they all had coughs, and their coughs would develop and worsen the longer the race went on, partly because the secretions in their chests were getting thicker.

Speaking to the riders and other experienced race doctors I learnt of the use of this medication, Fluimucil. A medication permitted by WADA, and popular throughout mainland Europe, it is commonly used as an over-the-counter effervescent powder added to a glass of water, in the management of the common cold and cough. When produced as a liquid for nebulisation, however, it's prescription only, and in the UK is used to break up the build-up of mucus in cystic fibrosis patients.

A nebuliser is a machine usually powered by oxygen to create a fine spray of the medication, which can be breathed in more effectively with a face mask. This is the standard method of administration for salbutamol in a life-threatening asthma attack.

There are two different types of cough medicine. Some that suppress a cough (Fisherman's Friends would be an example) and others aimed at making the cough more productive – a mucolytic such as Fluimucil would be an example of the second type. Using it allowed riders to cough and clear their chests when congested, bringing them a great deal of relief.

We introduced it in training, because it's preferable never to trial anything in a race for obvious reasons. The riders found it helped – most of them, at least – and that was that. The Brits got into Fluimucil. And I know that nobody is suggesting that Fluimucil is in any way performance-enhancing but it's worth saying anyway: it's not performance-enhancing. It's a legal decongestant used to treat a condition that was inhibiting performance, as is the right of the athlete.

At the time, you couldn't buy it as Fluimucil in the UK, so we got ours from an overseas pharmacy, which meant ordering it, having it delivered to the velodrome and then distributing it ourselves to wherever our teams were competing. It was Fluimucil in the infamous Jiffy bag delivered to the Dauphiné, a routine restock performed in possession of a French medicine import licence, which was a requirement for the upcoming Tour de France. On this occasion, it was delivered by a coach, Simon Cope, who was on his way out to us anyway. We often used staff as couriers if they were travelling, in order to cut down on costs. Something else common to cyclists is asthma.

The first thing to say is that asthma is a killer, so much so that every ten seconds in the UK, someone is having a life-threatening asthma attack. Three people will have died by the end of today from asthma, and two of those deaths were no doubt preventable had the patient's illness been managed more effectively.

So what is it? Well, it's a condition that affects your airways, causing difficulty breathing out. It affects five million people in the UK and one in ten children, and is characterised by sensitive airways that become inflamed (hence the use of anti-inflammatory corticosteroid medication) and tighten (thus the use of beta-agonist inhalers which relax the smooth muscle that surrounds the airway).

When you breathe in anything that irritates your airway, dust, air pollution – especially from vehicles – tobacco smoke, allergens such as animal fur, pollen, it causes the typical symptoms of chest tightness, wheezing, coughing and shortness of breath. Asthma associated with allergies usually starts in childhood; indeed, this is how we tend to think of asthma – as a lifelong illness. However, physical activity especially in cold and dry air can cool and dry the sensitive airway lining, provoking marked inflammation, resulting in the symptoms of asthma. This type of asthma is called 'exercise-induced bronchospasm'. You don't have to be asthmatic in the traditional sense to have EIB, and it's very prevalent in athletes. (Which is not to say that all wheezes are asthma, mind you. I managed a rider who had vocal cord dysfunction, and this was managed by having a speech therapist and a free-diving world champion teach her breathing techniques.)

Asthma is diagnosed using a spirometer, a computer attached to a mouthpiece. Patients breathe in and out, the software does what it does and flow volume loops are produced, with the key to diagnosis being a reduction in the speed of exhaled air coupled with symptoms that are variable, and that this observed reduction in air flow is reversible by a suitable reliever inhaler.

Effectively this means asking the patient to inhale an irritant designed to bring on an asthmatic attack, recording its effect and then administering a blue reliever inhaler (four 100mcg doses, which equals half a cyclist's WADA allowance for twelve hours) and demonstrating its reversal. This takes about thirty minutes and is done in every hospital clinic in the UK.

If an athlete with asthma symptoms takes this test and the diagnosis isn't for asthma then we'd probably move to EIB testing. The test for EIB is fairly unpleasant – as you might expect of something originally developed by the US Army.

The army couldn't explain why so many of their apparently healthy recruits were getting breathless on exertion, and so devised the eucapnic voluntary hyperventilation test (or EVH for short). The patient was asked to breathe air that contained 5 per cent carbon dioxide (vastly increased from the normal 0.04 per cent) at maximal breathing rates, and then asked to exercise to exhaustion for six minutes of increasing workload on a treadmill or cycle.

If the spirometer confirmed airway obstruction – in other words if an asthmatic attack had been induced – then the diagnosis of EIB could be made.

Once the diagnosis has been made the athlete can consider using asthma inhalers and other medication to protect the lung function from deteriorating during exercise. However, this does not increase lung function. It is not a performance gain.

There is now an oral treatment to help EIB, which incidentally also helps the more allergic patient, known as a leukotriene receptor antagonist. A further lung function test measures the concentration of exhaled nitric oxide (FENO test), which allergic airways produce in larger amounts. A result of over forty parts per billion suggests an allergic component to the patient's asthma. Analysis of a sputum sample for the presence of eosinophils (a type of white blood cell produced in an allergic response) is often positive but surprisingly hard to obtain due to the airway narrowing.

This is another example of the thoroughness of screening in professional sport. Not cheap, though. Gold standards cost money, though some would argue they help produce gold medals.

We did all of that for the riders at Team Sky, every year. They all had annual lung function tests, as well as the EVH test.

Elite athletes suffering from asthma or EIB are allowed, quite rightly under the WADA code, to take the medications that a normal asthma patient should be receiving; in other words, a preventer inhaler (the mainstay of safe and effective treatment) and a reliever (commonly known as the blue inhaler).

In August 2016, a computer hacking group called Fancy Bears hacked WADA and released their findings. Journalists spotted the fact that Wiggins had had TUEs for both salbutamol (blue reliever) and budesonide (brown preventer) in the past. Wiggins had a longstanding diagnosis of asthma; indeed, after his gold medal success at Athens 2004, he was interviewed for Asthma UK's magazine, and also appears on the front cover of their ten-year anniversary edition in 2014.

He's not unusual. The fact is that a lot of cyclists suffer from asthma in one form or another, not only because of the phenomenon of EIB, but if they have an inherited asthmatic tendency then it's much more likely to be exposed by the stress of professional sport than in normal life.

Callum Skinner, whose TUEs for asthma were also leaked by the Fancy Bears hack, actually published all his medical history as a child, which showed him in and out of hospital with life-threatening asthma attacks. No doubt about it, he is asthmatic. He needs anti-asthma medication to survive as a human being but also to be able to perform as an elite athlete, because those asthmatic symptoms will be exacerbated when he exercises.

Salbutamol, the usual reliever inhaler treatment for asthma, deserves a mention here. I know myself from having watched riders that they may well puff on an inhaler before they race, they may take it during the race and they may take it after the race if they're breathless or coughing, it's very difficult to remember exactly how many puffs they've had.

Factor in the dehydration that occurs during a race. Does that have an effect on the urinary excretion and concentration of Salbutamol? I'm sure it does, but robust scientific research is clearly lacking. The other thing to bear in mind is exactly what effect such a dose of Salbutamol might have. Clearly some drugs in the class of beta agonists to which Salbutamol belongs do have significant performance-enhancing properties but that's clenbuterol – a totally banned drug. Even so, common sense would suggest the time for Clenbuterol abuse to increase lean muscle mass would be in the training phase building up to a race. Not towards the end of a three-week stage race.

Incidentally, there are plenty of countries who have introduced Clenbuterol into the food chain in order to increase profit. Travelling to Mexico with the track team we were aware of the risks and so we took our own tinned chicken and ate local fish as a source of protein. That's how worried we were about ingesting Clenbuterol and testing positive.

And the irony of all this is that the current mood surrounding drugs and doping in cycling is a direct result of what I think of as the Armstrong Effect. But Armstrong himself? He never had an adverse analytical finding. He was found out through group evidence – whistle-blowing, in other words. Ultimately, of course, he confessed, but the net result was that it destroyed the public's trust in the analytical process. Now, personally, I can't understand how the analytical process didn't catch him. Was it due to analytical testing not being of sufficient quality?

Possibly, but analytic specificity and sensitivity is getting better all the time, and samples are stored for potential future analysis for eight years. I have increasing confidence in detection. But that requires more informed timing of out-of-competition testing and by all the national anti-doping agencies, not just in Europe.

14

Case Study: Bradley Wiggins, road and track cyclist

Four world-dominating years in the life of Bradley Wiggins

AFTER BRADLEY WIGGINS CRASHED OUT of the 2011 Tour de France with a broken collarbone, he tried not to dwell on it; rather, he did what he always did after any defeat. He looked forward. He liked to quote the Manchester United manager Alex Ferguson, who after a particularly heavy defeat would say that he'd prefer to talk about the next weekend's more important fixture. That was Bradley Wiggins's philosophy. He wanted to focus on the next one.

And so, in 2011, he began training for the following year's Tour de France. His aim was to win that, and then go on to win gold in the Olympics time trials.

Spoiler alert: he did both.

How? Well, I can't tell you *exactly* how, because obviously there was a lot of cycling involved. But I can tell you how he prepared, and where his asthma comes into it all.

So, in October of that year, he had been allowed a month off for what we call relative rest, which meant that he'd be riding on most days, spinning his legs, watching what he ate and drank and keeping an eye on his body fat.

Training began in earnest in November 2011, the regime supervised by a quietly spoken Australian sports scientist, Tim Kerrison, a very bright guy who had particular skill with data analysis and number crunching. In order to familiarise himself with the sport, Kerrison had spent most of the previous year travelling around the pro-tour circuit in a camper van that he called Black Betty, talking to people, assimilating the sport, its history and the major players involved. What he came up with as a result was an innovative training and racing plan for Bradley Wiggins. A list of elite riders required to support him – otherwise known as the *domestiques* – was drawn up and their training and race schedule planned to dovetail with his.

The training that Kerrison brought to the team was indeed very innovative. There were the normal types of training familiar to cyclists: Zone 1, an easy-going recovery ride; Zone 2, for endurance, long but easy; Zone 3, a tempo ride, feeling some fatigue; Zone 3 spiking in Zone 4, sustained at your threshold, legs hurting – close to the limit, or 'on the rivet', an expression in cycling meaning you're forward on the saddle and pressing in the pubic bone instead of the sit bones of the bum. It's an uncomfortable position that nevertheless allows for maximum power generation; Zone 5, close to VO2 max and producing lactate. More about this in chapter 20 on training.

Case Study: Bradley Wiggins

It was Kerrison's use of Zone 4 that really ramped up at the Majorca camp in January 2012. 'That's when I began *serious* training,' was what Wiggins told me.

Sure enough, training levels escalated, and with that I began to have concerns about over-training.

Now, we'll talk about over-training in more depth later, but the long and the short of it is that it can have a profound impact on an athlete, not just physically, but psychologically, and it needs to be carefully monitored.

That, then, was my job, and I kept an eye on Wiggins's health, looking for signs of over-training and its close companion, under-recovery – the latter being even more of a concern, in my opinion. (Indeed, Brailsford often would say, 'There's no such thing as over-training; it's under-recovery that's the issue.')

Wiggins's training stress scores were calculated by looking at the training data: a combination of not just the miles clocked up but the speed, the duration, the metres climbed, the power output through the pedals, the cadence, (pedal rotation speed), his heart rate. All this could be downloaded by him and the results displayed on our laptops wherever we were.

Put all that data together and it creates a score: 150 was an easy day, 250 a hard day, 350 is 'emptying the tank' – an expression you hear a lot in cycling. A good training week would have a training stress score of 1,000. It was noted that when he went to races (i.e. something like the Tour de Algarve), his training stress score was 500 and this was effectively a de-training week with decreased load and then potential missed adaptation. That was when the decision was taken to do less racing and more training under stress, such as the infamous and feared two-week training camp on Mount Teide on Tenerife.

When a rider is carrying fatigue in training, markers of fitness drop but then can 'rebound' with adaptation. Quite simply the fitness levels are now better than before the training block and the desired increase is known as super-compensation. The plan, therefore, was to enter the early season races in a fatigued state, which for Wiggins was ninety per cent of his capability, not the full one hundred. He wasn't trying to win these races (although he won Paris–Nice, the Tour de Romandie and the Critérium du Dauphiné), just sharpen his racing skills and team work, the reason being that training was more beneficial to adaptation than racing, and that when he backed off ahead of the Tour de France and refreshed and recovered – that 'rebound' effect we're talking about – then he'd be able to give a hundred per cent for the Tour de France – and that was what would count.

Meanwhile, the mainstay of Bradley Wiggins's training became a three-day block with a one-day recovery. I believe this was a game-changing approach to training for the Tour de France. Day one would be for EPD, Explosive Power Development. This was a training effect of 30 seconds of maximal explosive performance designed to build up lactic acid in the muscles, prior to entering a brief stage of SAP, Sustained Aerobic Performance, which was to be held for ten minutes in a typical racing situation, usually on a specific climb or gradient thought to be significant in the upcoming Tour de France.

This process enabled him to train in lactic acidosis and so to develop systems to clear lactate efficiently, whilst still on full gas (another good cycling expression). The effect of this training on his time-trial performance was extraordinary.

Day two would be pure SAP training: a five-hour ride consisting of a one-hour warm-up, then three hours holding sustained aerobic power. Typically, he'd look to hold 360 watts for the whole three hours. As for energy requirements, he would concentrate on feeding every half hour, with mostly carbs, some protein and then have a one-hour warm-down ride to complete the day's training. A 3,000–5,000 calorie ride. Day three would be a calorie-deficient ride to burn fat. This ride would last for seven hours with the aim to burn 7,000 calories while only supplying the body with 3,500 calories.

He's a tall guy. He's six feet three inches. He felt his most effective race weight for a Grand Tour was 72kg, going as low as 69kg when training too hard. The more muscle mass you have the more power you have; the more weight you have, the harder it is to get over mountains. It's something that elite riders feel for, and fine-tune their weight accordingly.

At his lowest weight he found that his power output dropped off (presumably as a result of lost lean muscle mass) and his immune system gave way and I can certainly confirm that he had multiple niggling performance-affecting infections whilst at that weight. I was very happy with his target weight which the coach, rider and myself had agreed should be between 70kg and 72kg.

In the 2011 season, he was racing the Dauphiné at 71kg. After that, he started to dip below 70kg but this had an adverse effect on his power-to-weight ratio, something which was very important but difficult to get right. When he was racing in the team pursuit subsequent to leaving Team Sky, he was deliberately putting on lean muscle mass in the gym and increased his new body mass target to 80kg. At the other end of the scale, I've looked after riders who crash diet just before a tour. As a result, they've suffered significant hormonal changes and have under-performed. I can't stress enough that not just in elite sport but normal life weight management is a gradual process. Yo-yo dieting messes with your hormones and metabolic rate, and I highly recommend it is not done. Weight control for the man on the street is a lifestyle choice, a healthy balanced diet with some physical exertion. Either you enjoy both, or it's doomed not to last.

Anyway, this third day would start with a half portion of a protein powder and a cup of coffee followed by refuelling every half hour with protein gels or bars, plus appropriate levels of rehydration. And carbohydrate free. After this long ride, Wiggins was effectively in a ketotic state, which means that his body had depleted its carbohydrates stores and had instead gone in search of energy from fat stores, as well as potentially starting to metab-olise his own muscle protein. Feeding after that day's ride was a large piece of salmon and as much green salad as required and then a protein shake prior to bed.

It was possible to lose between 300g and 500g of body fat in a single day of this calorie-deficient riding. To do it, Wiggins had to dig deep into that so-called purple zone in which the hard men and women of cycling seem to be able to exist.

Would I say it was healthy? No. Are there short-term health

issues? Yes, there are significant side effects: exhaustion, listlessness, irritability, difficulty concentrating and trouble sleeping. Are there any long-term health issues? No. Was it done with informed consent? Of course. It was coach led, rider agreed and doctor supervised. Incidentally, Wiggins would do much of this training alone in Majorca, paying a local guy 30 euros a day to drive behind him with a supply of chilled water and electrolyte drinks. (Mark Cavendish does the same but uses an ex-colleague, a road and track rider called Rob Hales who follows behind on a moped equipped with carriers for the vast amounts of fluids necessary to rehydrate during a training ride. Typically, they'd drink one and a half litres every hour, much more as the temperature rose.) Wiggins was never bored, though. He never used to listen to music; instead, he was aware of time passing, the power output, heart rate, the cadence of the pedals, and he'd be thinking about rehydration, as well as refuelling every twenty-five to thirty minutes.

It was particularly tough for him on his SAP training days, when he would be 'on the rivet', hamstrings stretched to the limit. Back screaming, legs screaming, lungs screaming. He'd deserve his massage that evening.

The fourth day was effectively the rest day, a light day of maybe a couple of hours on the bike, when he was allowed to refuel and eat, effectively what he liked.

Aerodynamics were never a problem for him, because he had a particularly low aerodynamic profile on the bike. This was thanks to having very narrow shoulder blades, very short clavicles, a relatively skinny upper body (he rarely worked his arm muscles in the gym) and the fact he was able to draw his head and neck in between his shoulders, like a turtle.

And then there was the event itself, the 2012 Tour de France.

Prior to the start, he had a pre-Tour blood and urine test with the rest of the team as part of the mandatory UCI health monitoring. He also had a pre-race blood and urine test every day he was leading the race, which was for fourteen days. For each of those days, he also had a post-race urine sample as the GC leader. He also had an out-of-competition blood and urine test on both rest days. That adds up to seventeen days of testing.

The night before each stage he would make his gear choices. He usually went for 53/39 on the front and 11/23 at the back for a flat stage, and 11/28 for the mountains. There was a marked focus on maintaining cadence, his chosen pedal revolution of 90 per minute, with regard to maintaining power, particularly on the hills, and not be over-geared. On occasions, he would use a compact front-chain set, 52/36, particularly on days with very steep climbs. He rode 177½ cranks for aerodynamic reasons not power, and used an Osymetric (oval-shaped) front ring with Speedplay pedals. Riders are all different and you must choose what suits your almost inherent pedalling style.

For rehydration, he took a mix of plain water and bottles with carbohydrate and electrolytes at a standard concentration made up for all the riders. As previously mentioned, attempts had been made to tailor electrolyte addition to the rate of electrolytes lost in sweat, which had been tested in training on individual riders, but it proved too complicated to distribute in the race and was abandoned.

Case Study: Bradley Wiggins

The musettes were the feeding bags given to riders during the stage, and they were tailored to an individual rider's personal requirements, as one rider in the team suffered from coeliac disease, so couldn't tolerate any wheat products. Bradley Wiggins himself used a mixture of protein and carbohydrate gels and bars and for a mouth cleanser chose our nutritionist Nigel Mitchell's legendary rice cake (simplicity itself, you can cook it anywhere with a rice cooker. The recipe is in the appendix).

Pre-stage, he would take a 'recovery drink', a scoop of protein powder. After the stage, he would take the traditional recovery drink with the same scoop of protein powder usually whilst waiting in doping control, or for the podium ceremony or compulsory media commitments, then back to the bus, shower, have any wounds dressed, post-race weigh-in or whatever else needed to be done and then, as soon as possible – certainly aiming to be within that golden hour (when your muscles absorb the most nutrients and when glycogen is replaced most efficiently) – endeavour to eat a meal of rice or baked potatoes with tuna and agave topping.

As for further recovery, he was a great believer in soft-tissue therapy and also liked manipulation, particularly of the lower back. Compression leggings without fail. We tried ice baths in 2011 but didn't seem to make a gain.

He enjoyed recovery smoothies with the evening meals, mainly made from fresh vegetables, anything from kale, broccoli and ginger. He aimed, in conjunction with the nutritionist and the chef, to take between 5,000 and 6,000 quality calories per day on a typical hard day on the Tour de France, to try and maintain a positive calorific balance. And muscle mass.

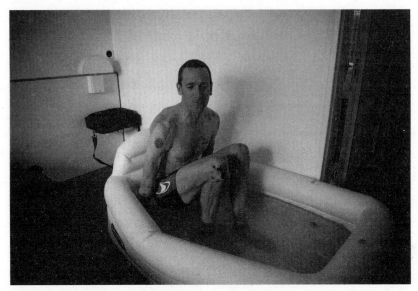

Sir Bradley Wiggins about to enter the ice bath in a hotel
bedroom 2011 Tour de France.

Supplements? They were pretty much limited to Omega 3 fish
oils (my prime choice for antioxidant) iron, either initially as the
high-concentrate iron water, later iron bisglycinate. Bizarrely (and
maybe it's that placebo effect) he was very keen on the antioxidant
pycnogenol, an extract of pine bark.

As always, I ensured it was from a reputable source, and we
checked the supply line. We tested for contaminants and, as I
said, it did no harm, but I firmly believe its effect was more
psychological than anything else. Antioxidants are thought to be
helpful in mopping up the harmful free radicals produced by
exercising muscle; other examples are vitamin C, coenzyme Q10
and beta-carotene.

Caffeine? He loved caffeine. Of course. A social stop at a café on a training ride, and a calorie-free drink. Wiggins would take up to 200mg of caffeine in the immediate preparation for a race, and within 20 minutes of starting, and the same dose during a lengthy time trial or day's stage racing.

His choice was, as I say, an espresso and a caffeine gel. A shot of espresso and a caffeine gel typically contain 100mg of caffeine each. Caffeine's role at this dose is mental alertness. The problem with using too much caffeine during a Grand Tour was that it also had a diuretic effect, causing you to pee more and negated attempts at maintaining adequate hydration. It also worsened the gastrointestinal side effects of the protein and carbohydrate feeding gels such as nausea, bloating and diarrhoea. More worrying though is that there are concerns of cardiac arrhythmias with very high levels in extreme exercise.

When I came to pro-cycling, it was almost obligatory to have a small can of 'full fat' Coca-Cola in the finish bag for the rider to drink and I can understand why: it was fizzy, refreshing and helped riders to rinse their palate from the various gels taken during the previous six hours of racing.

However, carbonated drinks with caffeine are no friend to digestive health, and I was able to persuade Wiggins and other Team Sky riders and British Cycling road riders to stop this ritual and rely on water at the finish.

And that was it. As I say, there was a fair bit of cycling involved, but the long and short of it is that he won and returned to the UK a different person in the eyes of the world. Prior to that he'd done well in the Olympics and had some success but that was really within cycling circles. He'd left home in Euxton, Lancashire, for the 2012 Tour de France a relatively unknown public figure, but returned a national hero.

Some years after that, of course, came the slings and arrows.

Which brings us on to triamcinolone.

Sitting here now, it feels as though Wiggins's name has been dragged through the mud. The two main allegations are that he was illegally injected with triamcinolone in the team bus after a race, and also that his approved injections of triamcinolone were given without due medical cause, in order to help with power-to-weight ratio rather than for his asthma and allergic rhinitis.

I'd like to take this opportunity to put some of that to bed.

Let's start with the allegation that triamcinolone was injected on the bus having arrived in a Jiffy bag at the Critérium du Dauphiné in 2011. We have already discussed the Alain Baxter effect, and we've discussed the need to have medications shipped to us. In a two-year period there was a large amount of different medications shipped out to various parts of the world, and as I've said, most of them came in Jiffy bags, so why that particular one should have been singled out for suspicion I'm not sure. As already mentioned, the Jiffy bag contained a routine restock of Fluimucil, not triamcinolone, requested from Phil Burt, the British Cycling physiotherapist back at the Manchester HQ. There was no injection in the back of the bus. I didn't have any medical reason to inject him, had no WADA-approved TUE to allow injection and would not have done so. And as you can imagine the back of the bus is a very public area after a race, it's full of riders, showering, rushing to get cleaned up and head home.

There have been some ghastly personal circumstances – the theft of my laptop, an ill-timed bout of ill health – that have prevented us being able to put the Jiffy bag and bus-injection tale to bed where it should be.

UK Anti-Doping had launched an investigation into the contents of the Jiffy bag, but the medical records that would have backed up our assertion that the envelope contained Fluimucil were on my laptop, which was stolen from my hotel room while I was on holiday in Santorini in August 2014. It was a violent burglary. The patio door glass was smashed and the hotel safe ripped from the wall. My passport was taken as well – leading to an extraordinarily stressful three days securing a police report, then being transferred to Crete for consular assistance.

I cooperated with UK Anti-Doping in the form of two three-to-four hour interviews with them, both recorded, as well as something in the region of 200 written answers to various questions they asked throughout the investigation. When it came to appearing before the parliamentary select committee in February 2017, I was finding it very stressful, but I was prepared. Prior to my appearance I was being briefed by my advisers in Canary Wharf when I suddenly found myself unable to talk. I just wanted to cry.

As a result, my solicitor withdrew me from giving public evidence, and I gave written evidence instead, a nine-page document that can be read on the Department for Digital, Culture, Media & Sport website.

Nevertheless, I'm sorry to the chairman of the committee, MP Damian Collins, for my non-appearance. It transpired that I was suffering from severe depression that had been building for some time. There's always a straw that breaks the camel's back, and that morning in Canary Wharf was just such a catalyst.

It's a subject – mental health – that we should talk about more openly, and I applaud the work of the Royal Princes in doing so. I never shared my issues with any colleague until it had gone too far but we should be able to, and colleagues must not be reluctant to ask, 'Are you really okay?' and be watchful for the warning signs and offer help and support, while patients, myself included, should admit symptoms and access health care sooner rather than later.

I have regrets, of course. My administrative system could and should have been much better. The fact that consultations take place in a hotel room, or at a race in a fast-moving competition environment away from your desk is not an excuse for poor medical record-keeping. I urge all new recruits to the speciality to benefit from my very public failing in this regard.

I fully understand that the theft of my laptop looks 'convenient', but there's nothing I can do about that. In some ways what's worse is the fact that it exposed another of my administrative failings, which was a failure to back up my laptop. The hard drive was encrypted, at least, so no sensitive information fell into the wrong hands, but that doesn't obscure the fact that I should have ensured that there was a copy of those records. In the wake of this incident, British Cycling and Team Sky now use a secure IT system managed by an external resource.

One thing that was the subject of some misreporting during this period was our use of Dropbox. We did indeed use Dropbox, but it was never intended for use as a medical records system. What had happened was that in the wake of the tragic death of the *soigneur* Txema González (discussed in chapter 18), we decided to implement a system whereby we could monitor the health status of riders and staff in real time – literally tracking race doctors' work remotely. However, we were not convinced that it was secure enough to trust with material as sensitive as elite athletes' medical records (and whether it was or it wasn't, I really couldn't say. It's just that we felt that way at the time) and we continued to use our laptops. Dr Peters' laptop was backed up by his PA, Jeff Battista. As a technological dunce I'd been asking British Cycling to do mine. In retrospect, I should have pushed for it.

My medicines management strategy was not what it should have been. Again I regret that. Latterly, I introduced a medicines management policy in order to address the issues raised there, but this might be thought to have been too late. The resources were, suddenly, available where before they had been scarce. Even so that's not an excuse for poor medical practice. Once again, I hope all sports docs and professional sports organisations can learn from this and ensure the standards that patients and the public expect are met, whether finances are available or not.

And with all that said, I trust that the lack of substance to the allegation, not to mention the accompanying absence of a single adverse analytical finding, is enough to rob it of any credence. As we've said, Wiggins was tested day in, day out during the

2012 Tour de France. No prohibited substances were found in him for the simple reason that there were no prohibited substances in him.

As far as the second allegation goes, it's a matter of public record that Wiggins was given a TUE for three separate injections of triamcinolone in 2011, 2012 and 2013. Nobody's disputing that those injections took place before the Tour de France in 2011, again in 2012 and the Giro d'Italia in 2013. The problem seems to be the suspicion that Wiggins did not need those injections; that we at Team Sky were somehow gaming the system; and that while we may not have broken any of the sport's laws we were guilty of an ethical breach, and at the very least had broken our own in-house code as set down by Brailsford; ultimately, that we had crossed the line.

None of which is accurate, because although I didn't get involved with Wiggins until 2010, his asthma was already a matter of public record, and had been for years. I refer you to that 2004 edition of the Asthma UK magazine. As a requirement to compete at the Athens 2004 Olympics, the International Olympic Committee demanded an application form be submitted to use Salbutamol, which also recorded his medication for allergic rhinitis.

His asthma was also a known issue with the UCI. Up until about ten years ago, an athlete wanting to use a standard beta-agonist such as Salbutamol for their asthma had to apply to the UCI for a Therapeutic Use Exemption, and that didn't matter whether you were training or racing. Wiggins had been through that process, which involves the spirometry referred to in the previous chapter. He came to Team Sky with that medical record. There was nothing hidden or underhand about it at all.

Related to his asthma was the allergic rhinitis from which he also suffered. For that we tried him on different antihistamines. We tried one, it didn't seem to help. We tried another. All trial and error. We tried various nasal sprays, eye drops . . .

He had all the same tests, pre-season, as all the other riders did – cardiac and respiratory function tests – partly because it was good medicine, partly because some were a UCI mandatory medical monitoring requirement.

At the same time, we tried to work out why he was suffering more at certain times of the year. We did blood tests for allergy and he had a high overall score but he wasn't being affected by some of the usual things, house dust, cats and dogs, but pollen was way up high on the scale.

By now he was getting seriously frustrated. This was prior to the 2011 Tour de France and though he was on good form he was bothered by the allergic rhinitis. I knew that allergic rhinitis can exacerbate asthma. Riding in extreme heat had never been a problem for him. He was prepared for it; he'd done plenty of acclimatisation training, either on the road in Majorca or in the sauna that he'd had built in his back garden. As for the rain and cold, well, rain wasn't a particular problem, his *domestiques* were always ready with his rain cape. Rain was only a problem if he got cold after getting wet. Hard days in the Tour de France would involve climbing between 4,000 metres and 5,000 metres over cold and dry mountain passes at 1500–2000m elevation and this gave Wiggins problems because the cold, dry air found at these altitudes was having a cooling and a drying-out effect on the very sensitive mucosa lining of the airways, leading to an exacerbation of his asthma. Finally, the race covers 3500km in mid-summer through much of the French countryside. Beautiful to look at but no fun for hay fever sufferers.

So on 28 June 2011 – with the Tour de France due to start on 2 July – we took Wiggins to an ear, nose and throat specialist in Bolton, Mr Simon Hargreaves. 'Okay, Bradley, I'm going to put an endoscope up your nose,' announced Mr Hargreaves, and I sat watching a screen that gave us a great view of Wiggins's red, inflamed mucosa.

Now, we had a previous history of asthma as shown in his medical records. We had a present history of poor control of the symptoms of allergic rhinitis. He was already on six different medications: Ventolin inhaler, flixotide inhaler, Montelukast, levo-cetirizine, Avamys nasal spray, Opticrom eye drops. All at optimal doses. Mr Hargreaves recommended that as an appropriate next treatment step, a single dose of IM (intramuscular) corticosteroid should be considered. He recommended Kenalog (triamcinolone) at a dose of 40mg IM.

I knew it was a quick fix. I also knew it was effective. In general practice I'd given it to people whose attempts to sit exams or take their driving test were being thwarted by congested and dripping noses.

I have to say I was unaware of its alleged history of abuse in cycling. I did not know that it is said by some – particularly David Millar – to help riders lose weight without losing power. Personally, I doubt it has that property, and indeed, according to

Dr Brian Lipworth, of the Scottish Centre for Respiratory Research, speaking to the *Daily Telegraph*, there is 'no scientific reason' why a drug like triamcinolone would be performance-enhancing. He went on to say, 'An anabolic steroid like testosterone puts on muscle mass but this is a catabolic steroid which breaks down muscle. The benefits to David Millar were probably the fact that he was taking EPO and testosterone at the same time as he was using triamcinolone. So the anabolic effect of the testosterone probably counteracted the triamcinolone.'

Either way, I don't think any athlete will apply for a TUE for this purpose ever again. Hindsight is a wonderful thing. In 2011 UKAD produced a guide, how to apply for a Therapeutic Use Exemption for IM corticosteroids (in this case triamcinolone) for the treatment of hay fever and I've included it in the appendix.

The way the application goes is as follows. A doctor recommends a treatment; this is usually an independent consultant, as in this case. The team doctor then applies to the UCI using the WADA anti-doping administration system (ADAMS) medical for a Therapeutic Use Exemption to allow the recommended treatment. The application was made the following day, and I emailed the UCI doctor. After securing permission for a Therapeutic Use Exemption, I injected Wiggins with 40mg of triamcinolone, a perfectly normal medical dose – no matter what you might read elsewhere – carried out in Manchester before we left for France.

I went with him that year. In 2012, I didn't go to the Tour de France. In May 2012, Wiggins visited Mr Hargreaves again, and once more it was decided that, with the previous year's treatment having worked, we should apply for a second TUE for triamcinolone. On 26 June – four days prior to the Tour de France – he was injected again.

In 2013, Wiggins was kept out of the Tour de France because of injury. He entered the Giro, though – and was given his third and final TUE injection of triamcinolone beforehand – and I went with him to that. However, during the Giro, he contracted an upper respiratory tract infection.

I tried to treat him but he was coughing and his asthma was getting worse. His sputum turned from green to yellow. Almost certainly a secondary chest infection was developing. There was nothing I could do. So I said to him, 'Brad, I can't help you, I think you should withdraw.'

'I'm not withdrawing.'

Brailsford arrived. 'Oh, come on, Doc, try another day.'

I said, 'No, he's sick.'

The next morning, I dragged myself out of bed, for a pre-arranged dawn review only to discover that Wiggins had had an even worse night. 'That's it, he's not going on.'

And with that, he had to withdraw.

Wiggins, however, was able to recover as all successful athletes have to do after illness or injury. What makes Wiggins exceptional is that through appropriate training and adaptation he was able to switch between cycling disciplines and after leaving Team Sky returned to the track.

The Hour Record on 7 June 2015 was an interesting physiological challenge. He was prepared for it, and with the help of Heiko Salzwedel had tailored his training specifically towards that goal.

Case Study: Bradley Wiggins

The venue was the Lee Valley Velodrome in London, the Olympic track, and the date was chosen because historically it was always a warm summer's day, and anyone involved in cycling understands the critical importance of environmental conditions on aerodynamic drag. World records are broken on hot sunny days for the same reason that they're broken at altitude – the air is thinner, hence the aerodynamic drag is less.

However, the air pressure was much lower than predicted so that was against him. We had planned an optimal race temperature of 28 degrees but it was going to be higher than that and we knew there'd be a problem with cooling because the design of the aerodynamic helmet allowed for no cooling vents while the type of material in the skin suit, gloves and race socks would not be beneficial to losing temperature through sweating. He was well prepared, producing 1,200 watts off the line and attempting to hold 450 watts for the hour.

Unfortunately, we were unable to control the environment in the velodrome and it rose to 33 degrees, no doubt due to the fact that there were 5,000 excited, cheering people in there generating a lot of body heat. I watched him closely lap after lap. With 18 minutes to go he wobbled. He was in difficulty. I thought, *He's overcooking it, maybe going to drive himself to collapse.* Instinctively I grabbed my emergency bag . . .

But he did it. And he still holds that record. 54.526km, 33.88 miles.

And I sincerely hope that that is his legacy. Not all this other stuff, these anonymous allegations. I hope that the man on the street will not conclude that there is no smoke without fire (because in fact there is no fire). I hope that his legacy is that he is the only rider to win the Paris–Nice, the Tour de Romandie, the Critérium du Dauphiné, the Tour de France, and the Olympic time trial in a single season. I hope it's the fact that he's the only rider to win world and Olympic championships on track *and* road. I hope it's all those other achievements besides. The fact that he did it. And he did it according to those first principles. He did it without crossing the line.

I have cared for Wiggins on the track, on the road and at the Hour Record. He's always trained hard and listened to his coach. He's over-trained, under-recovered, been ill, been injured. But always honest, never looking for any performance advantage from his doctor, accepting advice and opinion from myself and my colleagues. Challenging to work with, funny, a pain in everyone's ass and he's certainly made some enemies.

But his legacy has been earned.

15

A Day in the Life (part two)

*From the end of breakfast to the race itself – sports science
playing its part every step of the way, every turn of the pedal*

THE RIDERS FINISH BREAKFAST, and then either see a soft-tissue masseur, a physiotherapist or me, to get their dressings changed. Then it's off to their rooms to pack – although of course they never carry their bags downstairs, all in the name of conserving energy.

Now they're gone I look around at the room that has been my bedroom but also the makeshift medical station for the duration of our one-night stay.

Riders have bled in this room. A bin is full of stained dressings for appropriate disposal. It looks like a crime scene. Later the hotel will need to be reimbursed for the towels we've ruined.

Downstairs in the lobby, and talk is of cycling now. Last night, the riders and coaches discussed such things as gear selection, chain rings and tyre pressure, and the mechanics stayed up late setting up the bikes on that basis. They would have worked even later if there had been a crash, when frames crack and a new bike will need making up to a specific fit from scratch.

Meanwhile, if a rider's changed his mind about his gear selection overnight, an exhausted mechanic will have to miss breakfast in order to tend to his whim.

Riders and mechanics have an interesting, sometimes complex relationship. Most riders treat their mechanics with the utmost respect. Some, however, are never satisfied, forever requesting extra fine-tuning or fettling – the seat height, usually. I call them the micro-adjusters.

Others, like Geraint Thomas, are the opposite. He once rode half a stage on another rider's bike, which had been given to him in error from the roof rack of the race car during a bike change. He just got on with it.

The long and the short of it is that the mechanics are excellent and take immense pride in their trade. Bike failures, known as 'mechanicals' are very rare.

We consult our phones. Riders and staff are provided with a schedule on WhatsApp. It tells us what time the bus leaves, when the race presentation will take place, what time is signing-on at the stage, what time the race starts.

Today the bus leaves at 9.15am. It's a pretty magnificent beast, the Death Star. It's designed around the riders, with the lion's share of space devoted to their extraordinary seats, which virtually double as beds. The seats go back, the footrest comes up; the riders are almost horizontal – an aspect that makes the Death Star truly innovative.

Also in the Death Star: a double shower, kitchen, washing machine and tumble dryer, compression boots and trousers, ice compression cuffs, nine riders, the doc, the physio, the swannies, the *directeur sportif,* and the boss. It's a tight fit, and there's not much privacy although we all do our best to give each other some personal space.

Anyway, we all troop on. And here's another Brailsford detail. He has the swannies make up nine two-litre drinking bottles of pineapple juice and water, and place them on the riders' seats so that each rider has to pick up his bottle before he's able to sit down and, as a result, is much more likely to begin drinking from it.

There's not much banter at this stage of the day. The riders are deep in thought, maybe looking at their race programmes for the profile of the race, the flat bits, the climbing bits, or perhaps checking Twitter, Facebook and so on. At the same time, they'll be preparing their numbers, by which I mean the numbers that are attached to the fronts of their suits, pinned with quaint, old-fashioned safety pins.

Team Sky prides itself on the meticulousness of their preparation. Someone from the team, usually Tim Kerrison, will have been sent out to recce the day's stage and film the finish, because it's very important that riders know exactly what to expect at that point of the race. Why? Because this is the point at which they will have to 'empty the tank'.

This concept of 'emptying the tank' is something unique to

athletes. You or I, if we ran a triathlon, we wouldn't push ourselves to the point of damage; we'd back off, give up, exhausted. Our bodies and minds would shut off.

But athletes are different. You may have heard of stories of people finishing ultra-endurance events such as triathlons. They have pushed themselves so hard that they've used all their nutrients and blood supply to their exercising muscles, and because of that the bowel has become ischaemic and died and they've needed a colectomy. (Sport, as I'm always saying – is not always healthy.) Jonny Brownlee being helped by his brother Alistair over the line. Callum Hawkins collapsing a mile and a half from gold at the Gold Coast Commonwealth Games: both are examples of pushing their bodies to the limit. The body is saying, *Lie down*, the brain and other vital organs need the blood's fuel and to be cooled down more than the muscles need to work. The athletes are capable of overcoming this basic survival instinct, fortunately both turned out all right.

Anyway, for a rider to see the finish ahead of time is a psychological boost. It prepares them mentally for having to dig deep and empty the tank. And that, after all, is what they train for, because for a rider, preparing for a race is training for a race.

After parking up in the parcours at the beginning of the stage, the screens are drawn and it really does feel like we're on a Death Star. The *directeur sportif*, Yates, and Brailsford make their way to the front of the bus, where all eyes fall upon them and they deliver a PowerPoint presentation on the coming stage, as well as showing the film collected by the recon.

A Day in the Life (part two)

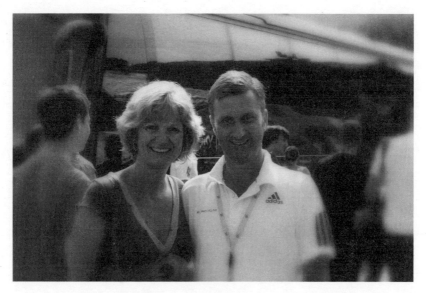

Myself with Frankie outside the Death Star in Morzine,
first rest day, 2010 Tour de France.

The presentation is slick and it covers tactics, pinpoints the dangerous parts of the course, the steep hills, the fast descents, the bad corners, and sounds like this: 'Okay, listen up everybody, today is stage four of the Tour de France. It's 189km, it's a flat stage, we expect the sprint teams to be dominant, there may be a breakaway, it's all down to the finish. We've got to conserve Brad, keep him safe, watch the side winds . . .'

On comes the film. 'Watch out for this roundabout, keep left, keep left there. If we're going to have a lead out, Eddie, you're going to be sprinter, we're going to lead you out, keep Bradley out of the way, keep him safe, watch him.'

This isn't word for word, you understand, I'm not listening *that* hard, but it goes a little something like that.

Now the riders go to the toilet and they pee for England after the two-litre bottle they've had to drink, not to mention the coffee. They're also in the habit of opening their bowels at the same time, losing unnecessary weight.

The trouble is that it's only a small toilet on a bus and the riders take a lot of protein supplementation, which creates foul flatulence, so it was often a pretty unpleasant place. Plus, it was often blocked. Ah, the glamour of life on the Death Star.

The blinds go up, the door is opened with a welcoming breeze and fresh air. The riders are peeping out, or nervously polishing their sunglasses or getting their kit ready.

Yates disembarks to see the press outside. Some riders are getting a little massage, some use fiery balm to warm their legs, while others just want a rub, and others want kinesiology tape applying. This is a relatively new thing. It's what's called a 'rehabilitative taping technique'. The elastic adhesive tape appears to improve function of the musculoskeletal system; it certainly relieves pain. It's unclear how it produces these effects and without doubt there'll be a 'placebo effect'.

So anyway, I'm called over to talk about this or that, discussing things with the physio, offering words of encouragement as they fiddle with their radios, adjusting the earpieces. They want a bit of tape to keep it from falling out. No, not black tape, it needs to be blue – the blue kinesiology tape, the blue of Team Sky.

They're getting their gloves, polishing their sunglasses a final time, turning their phones off, turning their phones on, checking their phones, sending something, turning their phones off again, almost ready now . . .

'Are we all ready?'

Wiggins is still getting ready.

'Come on Brad, come on Brad, come on Brad.'

'Right, let's go.'

They leave one after the other, clip-clip-clipping in their shoes to where the bikes are lined up outside, mechanics ready for last-minute alterations. 'Give me eight bar in the tyres,' and the mechanics do a little bit of fine fettling.

The riders have already selected what drinks they want on the bikes, and the bottles are kept cool right to the last minute. You don't want it left out in the sun, heating up or potentially contaminated by some villain putting drugs in it, so they are controlled and cooled, and we know exactly what to put on whose bike.

Now they get on their bikes. On go the sunglasses. Emotions hidden. Off they pedal, to sign on.

Race time is dependent on a number of factors, the defining one being the TV schedule. TV likes the race to finish at about 5pm. They work backwards from that, by calculating the projected speed of the peloton – that main group of cyclists in a race – meaning they'll arrive at the finish line at around 5pm for podium and press soon after. So sometimes we start at 10.30am. If it's a short, very steep mountain stage, we start at midday.

The peloton – that's what it's all about. It's like a living organism that looks after itself. It hydrates and feeds and stops for pee stops.

Riding in the peloton, on the flat, is a great way to save energy. The man in front of the peloton is expending 450 watts, but those behind only about 100 watts. This is because the aerodynamic drafting effect can be around 30 per cent, by which we mean that once a rider gets within one or two wheel lengths of a teammate, he may decrease his effort and energy expenditure by almost a third without a loss of speed. Riders in the peloton rotate to give each other a break.

Wiggins is worried about crashing and he prefers to be near the front where the risk of crashing is diminished.

Crashing in the peloton is a huge problem. When one goes down, often five, ten, twenty riders will go down with him.

It's the same story with amateurs who mimic the high-speed peloton of their racing idols, but often lack the bike-handling skills and awareness of what to do regarding potholes and other street furniture.

A colleague of mine who works at Leeds General Infirmary in A&E told me, 'It's the new weekend trauma. Instead of middle-aged men coming in in bike leathers, having crashed their high-powered motorbikes in the Yorkshire Dales, it is now middle-aged men in Lycra having crashed their expensive carbon fibre race bikes, having ridden in a peloton and come to grief.'

Back to the peloton, and its feeding needs are taken care of by our trusty friends the *soigneurs*. The *domestiques* swing to the side at the feeding station and grab the musettes, the little feeding bags mentioned earlier. They literally grab them off an outstretched arm, put the musettes over their shoulder, then catch up with the GC and other teammates and hand over the sustenance. Problem is, there are twenty teams all doing the same thing, hardly reducing speed. There's almost always a crash.

But it's so important, the refuelling. It's key to success. In order to avoid 'bonking', which is when you run out of energy supplies, you have to eat a lot during a stage race at the Tour de France. Every team has its own way of thinking. Team Sky has some very effective in-race feeding strategies.

We jump in the car. The one leading the race is car number one. So the order is this: the race director's car is at the front, then you've got the peloton, then you've got the doctor's medical car, two ambulances and then us, car number one.

And we're stuffed to the gills in this car. We've got nine bikes on the roof rack, a boot full of spares, cold weather and rain kit, mechanics' tools and drinks in a cool box. Inside we've got a TV, the Sky riders' two-way radio, Sky-to-Sky support radio, mobile phones, the race data sellotaped to the steering wheel, Yeats, who's driving, myself in the front passenger seat, a mechanic in the back. He always sits on the right. By tradition and for his safety the car always stops on the right. We're safer leaping out. So are the riders hurtling by, always on the left of the parked car.

Of course if you're car number one, that's great, whereas if you're car number twenty-two you might as well be watching it on telly, which is what they used to do.

The race begins in 'race neutral' for the first 3km. It's like a warm-up, very civilised, a gentleman's start, you might almost say. They're just warming up their legs, settling their breathing, perhaps calling for some last-second alterations to the bike set-up, in which case they pull over, their race car races up and fettles it and then they jump back on and they can soon catch up.

This bit is great. It's all great, but this bit is great in a different way, because it's in town, the crowds are gathered, kids are screaming, you get a real sense of atmosphere.

Now the race at the front starts to pick up speed and the riders follow suit. Depending on the tactics, some riders may jump ahead and get a breakaway. They get on TV but they rinse themselves so the GC's not bothered about that.

The radio crackles. Just static. A rider needs a new radio. From somewhere a spare radio appears and is handed out of the window to the *domestique* who's fallen back as Yates starts barking instructions at the riders. '*Okay, heads up it's a steep descent, you go past the church . . .*'

Yates is a great character. All that ever passes his lips is bread, red wine and olive oil, but he's as fit as a butcher's dog.

Sometimes a rider will come back for a bottle. There used to be a trick called 'sticky bottles' where a rider would supposedly be 'grabbing' a bottle from the *directeur sportif* in his support car, but the transfer would take just a little bit longer than it needed to as the rider benefitted from a little vehicular forward propulsion. Doesn't happen any more.

Me, I'm battling car sickness. I suffer from it terribly. Honestly, the number of times I've vomited down the Sky logo on the side of the car, and then had to get a bottle of water out of supplies and wash it off. I didn't realised I had to travel in a race car when

A Day in the Life (part two)

I signed up for Team Sky. It was something that came as a nasty surprise.

Because of it, I can't eat breakfast; it'll just come back up. I have to take anti-sickness tablets and I'm usually very tired because I've been up late and got up early. So at the beginning of the race and during periods when not much is going on I rest my head against the side of the car and close my eyes.

Can't fall asleep, though, not properly. I'm always listening out for problems on the radios, whatever they might be.

'Okay, heads up heads up, steep descent, sharp left turn at the bottom. Watch it it's skittish.'

Yates has all these great expressions. 'Shenanigans' is another.

'What the hell does that mean?' a foreign accent comes back.

'For fuck's sake, this isn't a radio station,' barks Wiggins, 'stop all this chatter.'

Not direct quotes you understand, but near as dammit.

'Crosswinds – crosswinds for five kilometres before the start of the climb.'

Problems might be mechanical. Riders will come back to the car with a fault, usually a brake binding, and a mechanic will lean out of the window of the car and try to fix it on the move. When this happens they're all allowed to hang on to the car whilst the mechanic is fettling – at great risk of losing his fingers – but it's fast-paced and exciting.

Sometimes they'd come back to the car for medical treatment for their road rash but of course they keep cycling so in order to treat them you have to lean out of the window and do it on

157

the go. It's fast and furious. You never know when the word 'chute!' is going to come on the radio. *'Chute, Team Sky,'* which means we're allowed to push to the front to deal with the broken bike, or worse an injured rider, never sure what we're going to find.

'Watch this descent, it's sketchy.'

'"Sketchy"? What's "sketchy"?'

Descents are the worst. Sean has the window open. He's steering with one hand, has a radio in the other, he's looking at the television, apparently unconcerned by the fact that we have a drop of hundreds of feet on one side of us and that we're in a controlled slide on a steep descent with riders ahead and more vehicles behind, each of which is also in a controlled slide and being driven by a maniac trying to do at least three things at once.

It takes its toll on the cars. We have a Jaguar mechanic who travels with us, and he services the car every night. We go through brake pads and tyres like you wouldn't believe. Wheels, too. We're always hitting kerbs. In Paris–Roubaix we once shattered a wheel on the fearsome cobbles.

A rider appears at the car window. He's dropped back. 'Doc, you know my knee. The tape's not helping, it's killing me. Could I get some painkillers?'

I check his knee as best I can. Dole out painkillers through the window. Riders are not allowed to cling to the car at that point but they're so good at riding without holding on to the handlebars that it doesn't really matter. The hard part is when they need a dressing. I'm not allowed to hold on to them;

they're not allowed to hold on to me. There's little I can do apart from spray them with antiseptic, attempt to cover the wound with a dressing held in place by the legendary 'string vest' Tubigrip and say, 'There, there, it's not serious. You can crack on.'

Riders are allowed to go to the official race medical car if they want – and they can hold on to it, too – but most riders will prefer to talk to their regular doctor. I only ever treat my riders, unless there's a medical emergency and the tour doctor or paramedics aren't available. In that case it's patients first, bike race second. The race car has left me behind more than once caring for another team's rider. Its an unspoken rule and the riders know it. It could be them.

A lot depends on the weather. Like Formula One drivers there are some riders who thrive in the wet, whereas others, like Wiggins, for example, don't like it at all, especially on descents. When it rained during the 2013 Giro he lost it, couldn't find the confidence he needed, and with Vincenzo Nibali attacking him on the wet descents he was a long way out of his comfort zone. That's the thing about descents. Some riders take risks, some attack, some people accept that they'll lose time, others just hang on for grim death and try to survive.

Ascents, with riders climbing, often for 15-20 km at average gradients of 7–10 per cent, is where the race is won or lost. It's my favourite part of any stage. It usually comes down to man on man. They look across at each other, sizing each other up and then one will put the hammer down and attack. The climbing bunch will crack, and riders will pop out the back, blown. Right at the back is what they call the *grupetta*, the back markers who are there either because they're rinsed or injured. Technically they have to make a certain time or be disqualified, but in reality there's often a bit of leeway involved, especially if the *grupetta* is particularly large. You can't go disqualifying half the field.

Some riders do well in heat, others fall apart. Sunburn is a problem, because the race jersey offers no protection – the fabric is designed for optimum heat loss. You need a waterproof sun cream, because they sweat, but of course they never reapplied it once the race has started; you just have to hope that their skin is already tanned enough. If it's very hot then you have to keep reminding the riders to drink, but that is about it; they can tolerate the heat. What they really hate is the wind. Head winds are awful because it requires so much effort to ride. Side winds are awful because the peloton assumes a dangerous 'echelon' formation where the end of each row pokes out ahead of the one next to it, with each rider trying to get in the other guy's wind shadow, and it all gets very scary. What most riders fear is one of those big high-speed peloton crashes that you see on TV where it's like dominoes. One goes down and the next thing you know up to twenty bikes are on the deck.

And that's when I get to leave the car. Most riders, if they and the bike are intact enough to carry on, will do just that, and many is the time that I've dashed out of the car, emergency bag in hand, only to see my rider disappear over the horizon. Equally, I've gone pelting through the carnage of cars, TV, motorbikes, officials, to find the mangle tangle of bodies and torn Lycra.

A Day in the Life (part two)

Rapid assessment, basic treatment, then back in the car, join the race again.

Once more, I lean my head against the door, with the constant chatter from Sean Yates in one ear, *'Ready? Five kilometres ahead road narrows, street furniture. Heads up.'* And keeping one ear out for trouble.

16

Cars and Bikes Don't Mix

Take all the precautions you can, but at some point you're going to come off (oh, and the real reason that cyclists shave their legs)

'*CHUTE!*' – THE RADIO CALL that us race doctors all dread.

The first time I heard it was Qatar, 2010, my first experience of being a race doctor with Team Sky.

Everything was provided by the race organisers, so instead of our own team cars we had huge four-wheel drive pick-up trucks, one for the race lead, the other for the second car.

Some bright spark had said, 'Doc can drive the second car,' and that was fine by me, pretty exciting really, and off we went, my first race. The peloton drew off, and behind that came the first team cars, including us, and then behind us the ambulance and the second team cars lead out.

I wasn't to know this at the time, but it was very odd to hear 'chute!' at such an early stage of the race. After all, we were still in the neutralised zone, the first few miles before the race actually starts, when the cyclists are heading out of town and to the race start. And then for some reason – and even he doesn't quite know how it happened – Kurt Asle Arvesen had crashed.

I grabbed my bag, jumped out of the 4x4 – 'Sorry, someone else'll have to drive' – and went to where he sat on the road, grimacing with pain and looking a little bewildered.

It wasn't bad. There was no trauma requiring on-site attention, but right away I knew his collarbone was broken. We bundled him into an ambulance and took him to a state-of-the-art Qatari private hospital, where I decided that it was best to get the collarbone fixed at home, booked him a business-class ticket, and left him with his arm in a sling and a supply of painkillers.

By the time I returned to the hotel, the stage was almost over. Apparently it had been blighted by terrible crosswinds, and there had been some bad falls, including our riders.

What followed was a steep learning curve, as I came across what is colloquially know as 'road rash' for the first time.

The following day I wasn't asked to drive, which was something of a blessing. As I was to learn during my time in cycling, driving in the peloton is a hazardous affair. You've got bike riders all around you, you're moving fast, you've got pedestrians stepping off pavements, other cars, the media. Personally, I think you should really be a pro bike rider to do it. Why? Simple things like anticipating what the peloton is about to do, knowing the right lines around corners, how to deal with hairpins.

And of course there are numerous incidents where riders have been hit by cars, a notable one being a Spanish rider of ours, Juan Antonio Flecha, who along with another rider, Johnny Hoogerland, were hit by a France Télévisions car on the ninth stage of the Tour de France 2011. Hoogerland was tossed into a barbed wire – an astonishing, frightening bit of film that you can see on YouTube. Both riders, amazingly, managed to get back on their bikes.

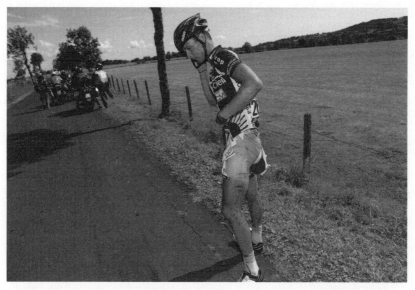

Johnny Hoogerland after being sideswiped by a France Télévisions car, stage 9, 2011 Tour de France.

We drew alongside Flecha in the team car. His jersey and bib shorts were torn to shreds and he was bashed up but otherwise unharmed. Treating him out of the car window on the move, I checked for concussion, cleaned the abrasion on his elbow and knee, applied antiseptic and a bandage best I could, while the rest of his extensive road rash would have to wait until back at the hotel. (And indeed, it was to be the worst case of skin loss I'd ever see.)

Meanwhile, his vision was clouded because he understandably felt robbed of a possible Tour de France stage win, which would have been a huge achievement. He was incensed, and really taking it out on the pedals. Fact is, cars and bikes do not mix.

Back to that second day in Qatar and it was like unarmed combat out there. Crosswinds were playing havoc again, massive potholes, too; riders falling like ninepins.

The first thing to strike me was that it was an enormous help that riders shave their legs. Funnily enough, when I'd first announced that I was going off to be team doctor for a bunch of cyclists, a few people had mentioned to me the fact that all cyclists shave their legs. It was one of those things at the time – the one thing everybody knew about professional cyclists: they all shave their legs.

'Will you be shaving yours?' went the joke.

No, was the answer. But on entering the sport I had certainly discovered that it was true. Whether they're using Veet or razors, they're all making sure that their legs are hairless.

At first I had assumed it was something to do with aerodynamics. That's how naïve I was. In fact, it's more to do with the soft-tissue massage afterwards, because when you're having soft-tissue massage on a daily basis, you get folliculitis, inflammation and infection of the hair follicles from being constantly rubbed. And that's why they take all the hair off, to make the massage soft and gentle.

But the good thing from my point of view as a doctor was that when they inevitably – and they all do at some stage – fall off and lose their top layers of skin, there's no hair to get stuck in the dressing because the hairs grow slower than the new skin.

I was learning a lot more about road rash. I was finding that it's not a 'rash', it's a skin abrasion caused by friction. What happens is that when a rider comes off his bike at 50–60km an hour on to tarmac containing dirt and all sorts of other contaminants, they lose that top layer of skin. The Lycra? It goes. It basically melts.

It can be difficult to deal with because it sometimes gets stuck in the wound but is otherwise not a factor in the injury. No, the injury itself is solely caused by the skin rubbing on the road. The friction on the road tears off the superficial layers of skin but also causes a thermal burn.

If you're an amateur the rash should be immediately rinsed, cleaned and cooled with lots of tap water. The pros, on the other hand, have to wait until they reach the bus, in order to have the wound cleaned. Personally, I use a Betadine surgical scrubbing brush, the type surgeons use to scrub up before surgery. You could use a soft nail brush and antiseptic. You must remove the grit. It's best done as quickly as possible because it's going to hurt; it's much more painful than a cut wound, because there are a great many more nerve-endings involved.

It was after Qatar that I began discussing this with sports medicine colleagues and a plastic surgeon, who agreed with me. 'No, this is basically a thermal burn that you've got here, you need to dress it as you would a burn,' which was illuminating.

From now on I would be using wound dressings for burns, where previously they'd used basic dressings which they'd pull off after a day, ripping off the top layer of healing skin at the same time. As a result, the road rash wounds were healing more slowly. It was like first aid medicine, no more sophisticated than that.

So I engaged with a company called Systagenix, based in Skipton at the time. I went to see them. They were interested in the fact that I was using their Tielle burns dressings in cycling; they'd only ever supplied them to hospitals before.

The dressings were fantastic. Having applied them to the wound, you could leave them on for two or three days at a time, which was unheard of in cycling but allowed the undisturbed and moist skin to re-epithelialise underneath, while at the same time drawing tissue fluid into the dressing, effectively cleaning the wound, so that when, two or three days later, you took off the dressing it would reveal almost a new skin underneath. Thereafter the wound is best left open to heal. However, this isn't usually an option for the peloton as it needs protecting from road dirt contamination. This is very important, because road rash on top of road rash is very common, and as painful as you'd expect.

I shared my road rash findings freely with my colleagues on other cycling teams because I don't believe that if you have a good medical idea, you should keep it to yourself. And after all, this wasn't a huge performance gain, it was about the welfare of the athletes, which if it isn't always uppermost in our minds then it should be. It's my belief that we as doctors should bring everything up to a level playing field; all doctors should allow athletes to operate at peak performance. As far as I know, most teams use similar dressings now, a big success for me – and one of those instances where I was able to bring medicine into the sport. There is an advice sheet on managing road rash and its complications in the appendix.

During the Tour de France, the doctor would always go in the race car unless it was a so-called 'safe stage', which meant it would be a sprint finish and you'd wait ahead by the line, or the last stage, when Brailsford, or an important sponsor or even James Murdoch himself would travel in the car.

In the race car we'd have emergency equipment. The ambulances in the Tour de France were very well equipped, which isn't always the case at other races, but in France, it was reassuring to know that the ambulance, race doctor and paramedics would be on the scene if not before you, then close behind.

Often if it's a crash the rider will have got back on his bike and left before either the race doctor or the team doctor has had an opportunity to assess the clinical situation. Concussion management is improving in a lot of sports, but it's not in cycling for this reason. And the fact is that it's a very concussive sport. You only need to look at footage of riders coming off at speed to appreciate that.

As it was, the riders would often be back on their bike and disappearing over the horizon before I'd had a chance to assess them. We would have to catch them up in the car and ask them how they were feeling (again, you can see footage of this in action after the Flecha crash, although you can't see me, I'm in the car) and I would do an assessment on the run.

The Line

These are hard men; they'll always tell you that they're okay to continue and you might be forced into making a decision that ends their stage. Good luck with that, Doc. It was something I was always prepared to do if needs be – if I diagnosed concussion or any other condition that would have worsened by continuing – but not something I ever actually had to do. Most of the time it's painkillers and off you go.

But that's the Tour de France, which has excellent medical cover, local hospitals who know you're racing in town and who remain on standby.

Where it all comes apart is when we go to different venues in different countries. I remember a particular event in Mexico, a kierin, where sprinters initially gain speed by riding behind a motorbike. A very exciting, fast and aggressive race.

The race was going full pelt, and being in Mexico, we were at altitude, so the riders were going faster than they were accustomed to. There was a lot of talk about there possibly being a crash at some stage throughout the day, and sure enough there was, a Malaysian rider, Josiah Ng, went down really hard.

At a track you can tell by the sound if it's a serious crash, and this was an awful thwack, the kind of impact you just knew was a bad one.

Sure enough, I saw his limp body slither down the wooden track and watched for signs of movement, hoping he might revive right away. He didn't move, and those little warning bells going off in my head grew that little bit louder.

Big warning sign when they don't move. Big, big warning sign. It's like watching a football game. If a player's down, writhing about and groaning, I'm not saying he's play-acting necessarily but you know he's not seriously injured, not in the way that a doctor defines seriously anyway. Because if he's seriously injured, he's immobile.

Ng was completely still. A couple of first-aiders had got to him quickly, sliding to their knees on the wooden track, one of them talking quickly in to a walkie-talkie. But doing nothing for the patient.

I'm glad to say that at times like that you go into a kind of auto-pilot. My trauma bag was in my hand before I knew it, and moments later I was on the track with two of our staff, who were used to backing me up.

A Spanish doctor joined us, a very good emergency medic who I subsequently invited to join Team Sky, and together, and in the absence of any other medical cover, we took control of the situation.

Which was: Ng was unconscious and not breathing. At that point he had a cardiac output, but if he wasn't breathing he wouldn't do for long. The decision was made to intubate him, which means sticking an endotracheal tube in his windpipe to help him breathe. It's a fairly simple procedure, and I had the equipment in my bag (a bit over the top, you might have thought – right up until that moment). It involves using a metal instrument with a built-in torch to keep the tongue to one side so that the larynx and entrance to the trachea is visible, after which a flexible airway (in other words a length of medical piping) is placed into the trachea.

We did that and then hand-ventilated him with a bag and

mask, maintaining his airway and keeping him alive, all of which is fairly standard procedure – something a paramedic might do at a road traffic collision.

We loaded Ng into an arriving ambulance only to discover that it was poorly equipped – little more than a means of transport with a red cross on the side. Worse was to come when the ambulance tried to leave the building. It's a pressurised dome with two doors that have to be opened one at a time in order that it doesn't lose pressure. Only, one of the doors wouldn't open, so we were stuck in the ambulance unable to exit the velodrome. It might have been funny if we hadn't been trying to ventilate Ng by hand at the time.

As it was, it wasn't funny – not at all.

I had a pulse oximeter with me, similar to that used in any hospital or trauma unit. You place a sensor on the end of the patient's fingertip in order to measure the partial pressure of oxygen in their blood, how much oxygen the lungs are supplying. Yours, now, will be ninety-nine per cent. His would have been less than that because we were at altitude, so the partial pressure of oxygen is less, which is why the air is thinner and why you race faster in any sport involving aerodynamics.

And as we monitored him, still continuing to ventilate him, he began to deteriorate.

Tachycardia, a bad sign. Falling oxygen levels in his blood, a very bad sign.

It was clear that he had what's called a tension pneumothorax, which means that he'd presumably fractured some ribs in the crash, and that had torn the lining of the lung so that it was inflating, but not deflating. In other words, it's like a balloon getting bigger and bigger; the lung gets compressed and presses on major vessels returning blood to the heart.

It's usually a terminal event.

Still there in the ambulance, the decision was made to put in a chest drain in order to remove air from the expanding lining of his lung.

I took deep breaths, trying to ignore the confusion around me. The velodrome staff were still trying to get the doors of the track open, the ambulance at a frustrating standstill as I found the plastic tube for the chest drain in my bag and glanced at the Spanish doctor, who gave me a reassuring nod.

I tried not to think about what I was doing – that I was about to thrust a large intravenous cannula into the fifth intercostal space in the mid-clavicular line just below the nipple. To the outsider it looks as though you're stabbing the patient in the heart but you're not, you're putting it into a safe space.

Well. You are – as long as it goes the way you want it to go. As long as nothing goes wrong.

But you can't think about that. You let training and experience guide you. And thank God my hands were steady as I punched the cannula into his chest wall.

The exact placement. There was the tell-tale hiss of air as the balloon deflated.

And now we held our breaths, both of us watching the pulse oximeter, praying for change. The difference was almost immediate. Ng's oxygen saturations increased, his tachycardia settled. He'd been moments from death, but now he was stabilised.

The Line

Later, I'd visit him in hospital. His injuries, a broken right clavicle, two broken ribs, a collapsed lung, haemothorax, huge skin abrasions. Even so, he'd return to cycling within a couple of months.

But for the moment we breathed huge sighs of relief, knowing that we were out of the woods. And at that moment, they finally got the velodrome doors open.

17

Case Study: Liam Phillips, BMX World Champion

We can rebuild him . . .

NG'S NEAR-DEATH EXPERIENCE WAS BIG NEWS in cycling at the time. What's more, it marked a change in attitude around medical cover at track events.

For a start I found myself more in demand as riders began insisting I join them at all track events. This is the doctor-as-talisman effect that I've touched on previously, a flesh-and-blood version of the placebo effect. Clearly I couldn't personally make it to every track event, but I did ensure that another doctor was always despatched with the team.

In light of what had been the lack of cover in Mexico, I got in touch with the UCI in order to discuss medical care at track events. I'm pleased to say that it began to improve from then on.

In the vanguard of this advance was BMX, which has always

benefitted from superior medical care. No prizes for guessing why. It's what you call a trauma sport; indeed, at British Cycling, BMX created more work from serious musculoskeletal injuries, fractures and concussion than all the other disciplines – mountain biking, track and road – combined. The BMX budget for orthopaedic surgery was sky-high.

The problem was that while BMX had begun on the forgiving red dirt tracks in California, it had moved into Europe, where they used concrete-based tracks and just as bikes and cars don't mix, nor do speed and concrete.

Oh, but there's more. Some enthusiast decided to change the start ramp used at the Olympic Games from 5m high to 8m high, now known as Supercross BMX, which increases launch velocity enormously. It makes it a more exciting spectator sport but increases the danger. It was soon the source of some of our worst musculoskeletal injuries, fractures and concussions.

Which brings me on to Liam Phillips.

A great lad, Phillips has got BMX in his blood – his dad is a coach, his sister races, and together they helped found a local BMX club in their hometown, Burnham-on-Sea in Somerset. By the age of five he was winning major BMX titles.

He spent a lot of time in the gym and was superbly trainable. For strength and conditioning nobody could touch him apart from maybe Hoy. Writing this book, I caught up with him and he emailed me some stats that may interest any weight-training enthusiasts: 'Regarding weights, my personal best squat was 215kg and trap bar deadlift was 285kg. My bodyweight was 84kg, my peak power on the start ramp was 2,600w.'

Case Study: Liam Phillips

And that, by the way, is impressive.

There really is nothing else like BMX. The public used the cycling track a great deal at the Manchester velodrome, but they flocked to the BMX track. For younger riders it's exciting, the helmets and pads are cool, and there's music blasting away. What's not to like?

At British Cycling, we had a shed of a building housing the UK's first indoor Supercross 8m start ramp, a structure so high and so scary that we introduced a rule whereby only athletes were allowed to use it. (This was *after* several members of staff fractured ribs and collarbones on the 5m ramp).

And what this track did was enable British Cycling to change the game by modelling their training course on the Olympic course, preparing themselves in training and producing some of the brightest stars in the sport.

And of all the bright stars, Phillips was the brightest. Trouble was, he was always injured. He had major issues with a crash in 2010. A fractured blade of the scapular (the shoulder blade), it was, which was an unusual injury – hard to diagnose and tricky to manage.

After that he became a bit wary of injury and instead trained as a velodrome sprint cyclist. The thing was, though, that his heart lay in BMX. He loved its daredevil, combative nature, and in October 2011 he returned amid great fanfare and heightened expectations for his performance in the 2012 London Olympics.

Phillips was driven, no doubt about it. The kind of athlete who needs protecting from himself. He'd pick up an injury but still want to compete and it was a constant battle with him to

177

see that he didn't do himself permanent harm. For example, he was frequently fracturing his wrists, a common injury for BMX riders who start from this tremendous, velocity-driven launch to being airborne and land with huge forces going through the handlebars and the concrete. They're also racing six abreast so there are six of them going for the first corner together. You might find it exciting as a spectator, but as a doctor I'm watching with my heart in my mouth.

Sure enough, Phillips broke his collarbone before the 2012 London Olympics, although we were able to fix it by plating. We rehabilitated him and trained him up in time to compete. He didn't win any medals, unfortunately, but I remember seeing him dressing before an event, and he looked like Spartacus, all strapped up, his body criss-crossed with operation scars.

But it never fazed him; he never lost his confidence or courage. He loved his sport; he was great to have around and a huge inspiration to younger members of the team – not just in BMX but in track and road, too. I can't say it enough: cyclists love a hard man.

When we were coming up to Rio, once again hopes were pinned on him for medal success, especially as he'd become World Champion in the meantime. Then, during a training race, he crashed again. Fractured clavicle, yet again.

We rolled up our sleeves. We knew exactly how to manage it, we knew the timescales, and we were confident we could get him training again. We got him plated.

It's a power sport, so our first task was to maintain his strength and conditioning, while at the same time keeping him away from the bike. As I've said before, you can't cheat biology. You can't make the two ends of the bone heal any faster. There's a new bone being formed; it's a biological process and sports medicine isn't clever enough to change that. What we can do is ensure that the repair process is as efficient, the alignment as perfect as it can be, but we can't do anything to increase the speed or strength of the repair.

So with any athlete, and especially an athlete like Phillips, it's a case of protecting him from himself, so he doesn't put himself at risk of further injury or even permanent disability, from falling on it whilst still training

But this was ten weeks away from the Olympics.

And Phillips was Phillips. He was desperate to compete and to win. And in his opinion he was in great physical condition: power, times, training, and he had racing form, everything.

What I knew, however, was that he was in danger of doing permanent damage to himself, especially to his wrists. And we come back to what I'm always saying about sports medicine and how it's not just about winning, it's about knowing when to stop competing, which if you have to make it, is a very hard decision indeed. For us, we think, *What's the bloody point in winning an Olympic medal when it comes at the cost of an irreparably damaged, unstable and permanently painful wrist? So what if you haven't got a gold Olympic medal, you're World Champion.* But the athlete will think of all that training he or she has put in. They want that gold medal; the coach wants the gold medal. They're of the mindset that they want to push, push, push.

So we were getting pretty damn used to how to manage his dislocations and fractured bones reliably, effectively and efficiently.

At the same time, there's no point being simply a good doctor and forgetting the fact that the athlete still needs to train. There's no point handing him back to the coaches pre-Games and saying, 'There you go, fixed his clavicle for you,' and the rest of his body's deconditioned and he's not practised starts, jumps and racing lines – he's simply not race-ready. This is one of the unusual facets of sports medicine. It's not just the doctor–patient, it's doctor–patient–coach. That's unique to our field. Imagine suffering a health-related problem and having your boss there for the consultations. It just wouldn't happen, would it?

But we got him there. *Again.* Spartacus Phillips.

So Phillips got there and he's, obviously, a hot favourite, very dominant, he was almost unbeaten in that Olympic year; but, as it was, he'd gone well in training in Rio, and then qualified in tenth place to secure a place in the quarter-finals.

Then it came to the first of his three heats.

Okay, riders, random start. Riders ready watch the gate. Beep.

The gate went down, the six riders hurtling down the hill, all aiming to reach the corner first.

Phillips didn't quite get there. I never found out how or why, but one second he was on the bike, one blink later and a whole bunch of them, at least three, were on the deck, with Phillips out for the count.

I'd been waiting by the start ramp with my emergency kit, sweating in the sun, hoping for the best but prepared for the worst, and sure enough, *bang,* so I was virtually first on the scene, only to find that Phillips was unconscious. So I began the recovery procedure, which involved immobilising the neck, ensuring the airway was clear. Now, this is crucial: you need to maintain the airway.

Case Study: Liam Phillips

Say someone is involved in a car accident. They're wearing a seatbelt but they're knocked unconscious and they slump forward with their jaw on their chest or on the horn. A first-aider rushing to the scene might say, 'Leave him, don't touch him, he might have injured his spine, wait for the paramedics,' but if you leave him then the victim is more likely to die, because he's unconscious, his neck has slumped forwards, he's closed off his airways, he can't breathe himself.

So you have to open his airway but at the same time protect the cervical spine, and the way this is done is with what's called a jaw thrust, and it's done, not by thrusting but by gently moving the jaw forward. This is achieved by placing the thumbs behind the angle of the jaw and gently pulling it slightly forward. At this point breathing should return to normal.

It's similar to a situation in which someone is said to have 'swallowed their tongue'. That doesn't happen. The tongue is attached to the jaw. But it will drop down and close the airway when the patient is unconscious and lying on their back. Again, you have to perform a jaw thrust to open the airway. Most people will breathe when they're unconscious, but what they can't do is control the airway.

That's why when paramedics arrive, they will protect the cervical spine but also maintain the airway. They put an endotracheal tube down, just as I did to Ng in Mexico; they place the victim on a spinal board so the cervical spine and head will be fixed and the airway already protected so that the patient can be safely transported to hospital.

As a procedure it remains pretty much the same unless they've got a massive haemorrhage. If that's the case, they're going to die whatever you do to protect the neck and airway, so you have to start dealing with that.

Happily, that wasn't the case in this particular BMX accident. Neither was there a need for an endotracheal tube. Within seconds of my arrival, Phillips regained consciousness, although I kept him immobilised because we hadn't cleared his spine.

Clearing the spine – in other words, making sure it was safe to move the patient – was the job of a big American guy who used to do the medical extractions at the BMX events. If you were to go online you can see pictures of the crash and the recovery afterwards, and you can see that guy. Easy to spot, he's the biggest. His speciality was the cervical spine and airway. He used to say, 'If it's above the collarbone, it's mine. Below it – yours.'

Which is what he did that day. And I handed him over. But by this time Phillips was conscious and talking. The big paramedic was skilfully assessing him. 'Any pain in your neck? Any pain in your arms?'

No. No.

'Can you feel your arms and legs? Can you move them?'

Yes. Yes.

'Any tenderness here in the cervical spine?'

No.

The big man cleared the spine. Off came Phillips's helmet and we helped him unsteadily to his feet and led him off the course and on to a waiting golf buggy.

The big man departed. The course first-aiders and other

officials drifted away, panic over. It was just us now, making our way back to the medical room, leaving the intensity of the crowd behind.

I had started my assessment. 'Liam, can you remember the race, the crash, me arriving? Can you remember where we are, the date?'

He was accustomed to the inquisition, having had it so many times before, and he supplied the answers – but he was dazed and groggy. What's more, he was complaining of a severe headache, pressure in the head and dizziness. There was a sense that the lights were on but nobody was home. Other symptoms I was looking for (that weren't present on this occasion) were unsteadiness, visual problems, ringing in the ears, nausea, vomiting, slow responses, and a distracted, irritable state of mind.

Even so, I had already witnessed a brief unconsciousness. His racing was automatically over. My examination simply confirmed more clues that concussion was present. Perhaps the biggest clue was that his responses were slow and sluggish.

This athlete, usually so keen to compete, looked beaten.

No two ways about it. He had concussion.

It's worth saying something here about the management of concussion, a topical subject thanks to publicity surrounding high-profile cases in American football, boxing and rugby.

In rugby, it's brilliant. First hint of a head injury, the player comes off and a head injury substitute comes on. That's good medical practice and that's good athlete welfare. It takes at least ten minutes to properly assess a patient for concussion. Respect to those trailblazing sports doctors.

Football? Not the same. You can't just swap out the player as you can in rugby. So in football you have to assess the player at the side of the pitch with the manager in your earpiece, screaming, 'What the bloody hell is going on? Get him back out, he's only banged his head,' which means you have to risk-manage the situation very quickly.

Sometimes you can watch a video replay there and then, which is a massive help because it allows you to assess the mechanism and force of impact: where did they bang their head? Did he appear unconscious when he fell down? Did he start briefly twitching or adopt a limb posture that suggests a serious head injury?

In all these sports, your athlete stays within reach. Where we differ in cycling is that, often, a rider is back on their bike and gone before a doctor has the chance to properly assess if they're at risk from concussion. You've got a situation where a rider can crash at 70km/h on a descent with just 300g of foam for head protection, a crash often not witnessed by officials or staff, combined with effectively no ability to withdraw them from the competition to assess for head injury. You very rarely witness the mechanism of their injury. You can't see how hard they fall, what speed they were going at the time. Invariably, you're hearing, '*Chute! Chute!*' on the radio in the race car, but by the time you got there, they're gone. There must have been so many cases of riders putting themselves and others at risk with post-concussive symptoms because they haven't been adequately assessed. It's even like that at the track sometimes.

The prime example of this was Tom Skujins's crash in the 2015

Case Study: Liam Phillips

Tour of California. Watch it on YouTube. He clearly seems out of it, stumbling across the front of bikes and cars.

Cycling has unique challenges but this issue needs addressing, starting with moves to train coaches and race officials.

A basic guide is in the appendix and I urge any coach responsible for the welfare of his athletes to read it; how many times are you with them with no medic being present?

So what is concussion? It's defined as the functional disturbance of the brain (with no obvious structural pathology shown up by current scanning technology).

In the real world this means exhibiting symptoms and signs that the brain is injured and not working properly. These are often immediate; most develop in the space of forty-eight hours but can even take up to two weeks to develop.

There is no specific treatment or medication for it, but complete rest – cognitive (that's no reading, looking at phones, TVs or concentrating) as well as physical – for twenty-four hours is essential.

The take-home message is that an athlete doesn't have to be knocked unconscious in order to suffer from a concussive injury requiring removal from competition. In fact, fewer than 10 per cent of concussions are accompanied by loss of consciousness.

Direct trauma is usually the cause, the force of which the rider's foam helmet tries to dissipate, but it can also be caused by rotational trauma and whiplash-type forces, which these helmets cannot guard against. I am concerned that the present foam helmets, useful though they are, can't control the forces generated in crashes. Children and adolescents are more at risk of harm as their brains are still developing. More research and development is needed.

But something is better than nothing. Happily, there is no debate regarding the need to wear foam helmets for cycling, regardless of the speed. Especially for the kids. Let's set a good example and make it cool to wear them.

It took the tragic death of Andrei Kivilev in 2003 to force the UCI to act in making helmets compulsory in competition.

Meanwhile, governments should not be waiting any longer to make helmets compulsory for riders on public roads. Head-injury protection needs to be further improved and standards of approval met by manufacturers.

Many sports collect and publish concussion rates, which has raised awareness and driven better management and in my opinion it's time that the UCI addressed their lack of data.

But anyway, back to Phillips. Poor old Liam. When I got him back to the treatment room he looked at me, and I'll never forget the expression he wore: that of a beaten dog. He knew. And I knew that he knew. It was all over. There was no more Rio 2016 for him.

His coach arrived. His partner, Jess Varnish, was trying to get in touch so phones were ringing. But Phillips just stayed still for a long time, wearing that same look, his shoulders drooped – so uncharacteristic of him.

I hardly even needed to say it. 'Listen, Liam, this is it. It's over.'

He closed his eyes, gave a sigh of relief, perhaps because the decision was out of his hands, closed his eyes and rested on the bed.

*   *   *

Case Study: Liam Phillips

We arranged for a CT scan of his skull, where we were able to establish that he didn't have a bleed or fracture. I was happy with that, but even so he needed monitoring for at least twenty-four hours in order to be certain he didn't develop delayed complications which is something you need to watch out for in all head-injury patients. Please read and act on the head-injury instructions given to you in hospital. I checked in on him that night, then first thing and he was morose, resigned, but, most importantly, okay.

Just over a year later, after a couple more crashes, I heard that he'd retired altogether. I can't say I was surprised. This is not a complete list of his injuries but it goes something like this:

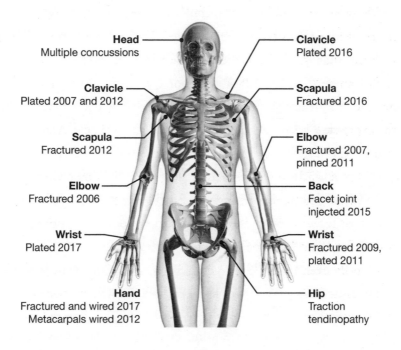

Head
Multiple concussions

Clavicle
Plated 2007 and 2012

Scapula
Fractured 2012

Elbow
Fractured 2006

Wrist
Plated 2017

Hand
Fractured and wired 2017
Metacarpals wired 2012

Clavicle
Plated 2016

Scapula
Fractured 2016

Elbow
Fractured 2007,
pinned 2011

Back
Facet joint
injected 2015

Wrist
Fractured 2009,
plated 2011

Hip
Traction
tendinopathy

List of injuries sustained by Liam 'Spartacus' Phillips, BMX Supercross racer.

'Elite sport is brutal for sure,' he told me recently. 'I remember from 2015–2017 spending half of my time receiving physio and treatment, and the other half training. So I spent as much time trying to keep my body in one piece as I did trying to get it bigger, stronger and faster. Madness.'

Madness indeed.

Some road riders were crash magnets, a term affectionately given to G – aka Geraint Thomas – at Team Sky. And the most common injury from falling off the bike is road rash and by far the most frequently occurring serious injury is a fractured clavicle.

As was the case with Wiggins, fractured clavicles were managed immediately and aggressively with internal fixation and early mobilisation, and the rider would be back on the bike within three or four days in a protected environment, in other words, a turbo trainer, or horse treadmill.

Apart from that we had lots of other upper limb fractures: the elbow, the wrist, the hand. More rare were severe fractures of the pelvis, lumbar spine and femur, but it's a high-impact, high-trauma sport, and so we ran the whole gauntlet of traumatic orthopaedics, fractured kneecaps in multiple pieces, fractured legs – you name it.

Track cycling is technically much safer because riders can slide without hitting anything too dangerous. No trees, no bollards. No cars. It causes friction burns, of course, and there are also splinters involved, which can be like arrows.

I remember Azizulhasni Awang crashing at the track World Cup in Manchester in February 2011, when he was taken to the first aid post, actually my medical room. I wandered in to take a look – only to see one of the biggest splinters I've ever laid eyes on.

Now, superficial splinters are a way of life at the track. Many riders, swannies or coaches simply pick them out. Myself, I had often removed deep, splinters using my portable ultrasound to assess the depth and location of the splinter, and then suturing in order to close the entry wound and allow return to competition.

This one? It was about 20cm long. It had gone clean through his leg. Both ends visible. I was fairly sure it was the only thing stopping Awang from bleeding to death. The same with any major penetrating injury: whatever is causing the injury, you leave it in place.

I glanced at the coach, an Australian, John Beasley, catching an almost imperceptible shake of his head and thought, *Crikey, that's big, right in tiger country*, and pulled rank: my medical room, my patient.

Right away, I transferred Awang to my local trauma centre. It was two days before an appropriately skilled vascular surgeon was available, who removed a splinter, which was just nicking the major tibial artery, its presence preventing a massive haemorrhage.

The main asset of an experienced doctor in any major trauma incident isn't just that they take control of the situation; they create calmness to allow rational thinking and coordinated action.

They know when complex life-saving surgery is required.

I was always terrified of a rider leaving the track. Thankfully

I only ever encountered one instance of this, when looking after a rider who left the track. His pedal had snapped off and the spindle pierced his arm and lacerated his brachial artery.

I was one of those on the scene for that, and it could have been really nasty. But fortunately for all concerned the artery went into spasm, didn't bleed excessively and blood loss was easily controlled with a tourniquet before he was taken to hospital.

However, you'd be wrong to think that trauma provided most of my workload; most of my time was spent dealing with the most common cause of musculoskeletal complaint in sports and that's overuse injury. The result of repetitive strain on the body in cycling particularly created problems with the knees, one being retro patellar knee pain. The patella articulates on two facets separated by a groove at the lower end of the femur (thigh). This joint is particularly compressed and thus potentially overloaded and damaged when the knee is bent.

Of course this happens ten of thousands of times a day in a long ride, and is a pain behind the kneecap that gets worse with increasing activity. Paradoxically, simply sitting with the knee bent for several hours can cause the pain. The Americans have a lovely term for this: 'moviegoer's knee'. So get up and stretch out.

Most cyclists will recognise this pain. An MR scan isn't much help, it just confirms inflammation on the joint surface. Overuse injury has many causes: too much or too intense exercise, especially if it's ramped up rapidly, but also muscles controlling joint movements may be fatigued, weak or injured, tissues around the joint may be too tight or too lax – all contributing to abnormal movement and therefore risk of harm. This is known as abnormal biomechanics.

Case Study: Liam Phillips

How to treat it? You have to look at the whole rider. Why is he or she getting it? Have they neglected their stretching and recovery? Over training on the bike or in the gym? Have their cycling shoes or cleats changed? Pedals too? Has their saddle position, saddle height, crank lengths or handlebars been altered?

So it was always a multifactorial analysis, drawing in the physiotherapist, soft-tissue therapist, strength-and-conditioning coach and of course their own coach. (Their own coach is always involved in sports medicine). That's what performance medicine was. It was getting all those ideas together in order to come up with a strategy.

There would initially be the usual first-aid management, relative rest, maybe ice cuff compression and strapping to off-load the joint. Maybe it would start with soft-tissue therapy to release any tightness affecting knee function. Rehab of muscle strength and coordination in the gym. Maybe a bike fit, maybe a discussion with the mechanics especially with the introduction of new bikes and kit.

But medicine is all about pattern recognition and certainly retropatellar pain – patellofemoral syndrome, as it's sometimes known – was our bread and butter and came with certain instantly recognisable patterns. The more experienced I became, the easier it was to spot them.

Unlike in football, muscle tears were rare and tended to happen in the gym when riders were lifting weights, but they were relatively easy to manage because muscles are very vascular, by which I mean they've got a great blood supply, and so tend to heal quickly.

However, if the tear involves the tendon which attaches the muscle to bone it will heal less efficiently and much more slowly, as it has a much poorer blood supply. MR scanning is most useful in determining the location and size of the tear, and helped me predict when the athlete can return to training.

Which brings us on to something we call 'return to play decisions'. In football it's a fitness test, in cycling it's called best judgement. Sometimes I had to take a calculated risk with the informed consent of the patient and knowledge of the coach. Often it depended how important it was to get the rider back and what their goal was.

It was easy in football. You had reserve players. You could even buy another one. 'Strength in depth' as they were always saying. But in British Cycling, athletes were thin on the ground. You can't buy riders in a national sport like British Cycling, you had to train them and progress them in the system. (Or lure them from other sports, rowing being a fertile hunting ground as mentioned earlier.)

We didn't have an unlimited number of endurance riders to throw in team pursuit at that level, especially as many graduate to the more lucrative road racing. We certainly didn't have an unlimited number of world-class sprinters. We really had to look after what we had and we all knew that, including the coaches who respected the fact that the riders needed to be looked after. And I'm pleased to say that's exactly what we did.

18

Hidden Dangers

Much of my job involved safeguarding against invisible threats . . .

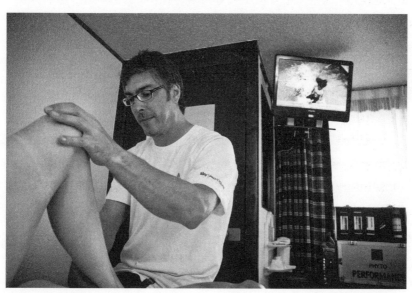

Txema González, perfect gentleman, family man and *soigneur*. 1967–2010.

TXEMA GONZÁLEZ WAS A FORTY-THREE-YEAR-OLD Spanish *soigneur*, a family man who was a great swanny to Wiggins. At the Vuelta a España in 2010 he started complaining of flu-like symptoms. A short time later, he was dead.

It turned out that he'd cut himself, a seemingly insignificant scratch on his leg but he'd contracted a bacterial infection and he'd died of sepsis.

In the wake of this awful incident, I began to think very seriously about sepsis, which, without wanting to sound overly dramatic, is the deadliest killer you've never heard of, and needs early diagnosis. I apologise that it doesn't have much to do with cycling but Txema's death was tragic and I want to take this opportunity to explain it and hopefully prevent someone else's early death.

Now, for a rider coming to me feeling generally 'unwell', it could mean a number of things: a minor upper-respiratory tract infection (which is, in fact, not at all minor to an athlete but very major indeed); a moderate attack of gastroenteritis (ditto) or in the worst-case scenario, full-blown flu, which is the end of the race for the cyclist. It's off to bed for you.

The fact is that a rider on Grand Tour suffers massive physiological and psychological stress, and this can contribute to immune system dysfunction, making them more susceptible to minor illnesses on exposure. So members of staff feeling unwell with these or other symptoms are asked to inform the doctor.

In all of these situations, the medic would advocate isolation and time away from other riders in addition to whatever else was prescribed. As well as that, the patient should of course be properly monitored – being especially vigilant for the development of sepsis.

Which is? A killer, as we've said. Forty thousand deaths a year in the UK. More than bowel, breast and prostate cancer combined.

And what's especially frightening about it is how deadly it is. A 30 per cent mortality rate by the time of admission to intensive care. Not to be confused with blood poisoning – that's septicaemia – it's a condition that arises when the body's immune system overreacts to an infection, essentially an allergic reaction to infection, causing extensive damage to the major organs. It can be caused by viral or fungal infections, but bacteria is by far the commonest cause.

Nevertheless, the real problem is the way it presents, because it will often appear to start with symptoms like flu, gastroenteritis, a urine infection or chest infection, which makes it very, very difficult to spot.

Risk factors, especially those relevant to cycling, are recent trauma, cuts and abrasions – and the resulting risk of an infection. This was the case, tragically, with González: a simple scratch to the leg that became infected. Meanwhile, in the general population, you must be careful to monitor the patient, especially the very frail, those over seventy-five years old, or babies under one years old, and you should look for the warning signs of very high fever, or – paradoxically – very low fever and/or a very rapid heart rate. If the patient *also* displays any one or more of the symptoms in this mnemonic then you should seek medical help right away:

S – slurred speech, confusion, lethargy.

E – extreme shivering and/or muscle pain.

P – passing very little or no urine in twenty-four hours.

S – severe breathlessness.

I – it feels like you're going to die (the patient will disclose this – listen to them).

S – skin mottled or discoloured, cold to the touch, or a rash that doesn't fade on compression with a drinking glass. Purplish lips.

Please phone for medical help and say, 'Could this be sepsis?'

The Zika virus was a nightmare at the Rio Olympics in 2016, for the simple reason that there were an awful lot of rumours circulating, a tremendous amount of anxiety generated, but very little in the way of actual facts. All we knew was that it was a mosquito-borne virus, almost certainly associated with serious birth defects, babies born with abnormally sized heads and under-developed brains, and that it was also associated with Guillain-Barré syndrome, a rare neurological disorder that can result in paralysis and death.

Of course we had a lot of female riders who were of reproductive age and in relationships, who were thinking, *I'll make it to the Olympics, then I'll have a year off and have a baby.* Or, *I'm going to finish cycling and have a family.*

So there was a lot of anxiety prior to going out there, and we looked into anti-mosquito sprays, nets, zappers, you name it. There wasn't a vaccine for it, unfortunately, but I oversaw other travel vaccinations – they're allowed by WADA – and this was one of those occasions where I managed to convince the majority of them to go for the full set. Some athletes didn't want travel vaccinations in case it affected their adaptation or performance or because they might get the rare side effects, but talk of the Zika virus had proved worrying enough to override most of their concerns.

The males in our party weren't especially concerned about the virus, but the women were. You have never seen so many people apply so much anti-mosquito cream in your life. I don't think any of them had a single bite the whole time they were out there. They rarely went outside unless they had to go and eat or race. Neither did they use the dozens of swimming pools the Brazilians had thoughtfully installed in the village for use after finishing a competition. They took this risk with potentially profound consequences very seriously. I was extraordinarily proud of them.

Arriving home, I advised they shouldn't try to conceive for six months afterwards. National guidance was conflicting and anyway not based on rigorous evidence.

There were some who were very disappointed by that. I was being badgered for blood tests, but I didn't have direct access to the NHS screening facility at Porton Down. That was reserved for those returning with full-blown flu and other symptoms.

Instead, I gave them what information I could and advised caution, which considering the potential impact of a Zika-infected pregnancy was the best option.

But if we're talking about hidden dangers, then I must discuss cardiac screening.

In a way, this story goes back to when I was a general practitioner in rural Lancashire.

Back then the ambulance service wasn't as advanced as it is now – they weren't much more than a medical transport service – so country doctors were often the first line of defence for cardiac arrest, collapse, diabetic emergency, epilepsy, road traffic collisions, people falling out of trees, cutting their legs off with chainsaws – whatever – and as result we were well equipped with emergency kit.

Personally, I found this part of the job both very intense, but also very rewarding, knowing that thanks to my medical training, I could help people with life-changing conditions from accident or illness, there and then.

I also carried a defibrillator and various other emergency cardiac drugs.

One Christmas, I was driving from the surgery home and there was a commotion at the traffic lights. A man had collapsed. Already on the scene was one of the nurses from the practice, who was doing cardiopulmonary resuscitation (CPR, and we'll talk about CPR in more detail shortly), so I stopped, and she continued with mouth-to-mouth ventilation and chest compressions as I prepared the defibrillator and shocked him.

Unfortunately, there was nothing we could do to save him. Not everyone who's had a heart attack responds to defibrillation, but it's always a possibility and time is of the essence – every minute that passes decreases the patient's chance of survival by 10 per cent.

A rather tragic tale, actually. It turned out that he'd left home in order to take Christmas presents to his grandchildren, but having got on the bus realised that he'd left the gifts at the bus stop. He'd got off at the next stop and was rushing back to claim them but unfortunately the exertion at his age was too much for his heart and he had a heart attack.

That was the background. And it meant that when I went into sports medicine I arrived with a good background in emergency medicine (which was to prove invaluable during the Josiah Ng incident).

So, when I went into sports medicine, I was well prepared. I'd attended courses on advanced life support and serious trauma. On one of the courses we were shown a clip of a seventeen-year-old girl, Claire Crawford, playing volleyball at an American high school. Suddenly she collapsed right there on the court.

Now, people should never – ever – collapse unconscious during exercise. If you're fit and healthy before you go on that pitch but you collapse, you haven't simply fainted through exertion, there's something seriously wrong.

But as this girl went down, the teachers recognised the danger and one of them rushed for the emergency defibrillator which hung in the sports hall, while the other dialled 911 to summon the paramedics.

They immediately defibrillated her, she regained consciousness and the paramedics came and whisked her away – all within the space of about fifteen minutes. The whole event was captured on a spectator's video. It is quite extraordinary viewing and it had a profound impact on me. Please go and look at the video for yourself. Look for 'Project S.A.V.E. Claire's story' on YouTube. You'll see that the charity equips schools and train teachers ready to use defibrillators in such events.

But if that had happened in Lancashire? I think they might have just said, 'Leave her; she's just fainted. Would our teachers have the skills for basic CPR? The equipment to defibrillate?

Some schools do. But there are many that don't, and this is something I'd like to change first in Lancashire, and then hopefully one day throughout the UK, by linking up with the local charity, Danstrust.

Danstrust began in the wake of the tragic death of a twenty-six-year-old lawyer, Dan Bagshaw, who suffered sudden cardiac death while running a marathon. Launched by his parents Peter and Shelagh Bagshaw the charity very kindly funded a cardiac screening session for the British Cycling podium squad and they are fundraising for this to happen in our local schools.

I strongly feel all schools and all organised sports should have coaches trained in CPR and equipped with defibrillators.

Then there was the case of Khalilou Fadiga, a player at Bolton Wanderers. A Senegalese international, Fadiga had played for Inter-Milan but then was released when it was discovered that he had an abnormal heart rhythm.

As far as I know, he considered retirement at that stage but decided against it; instead, he ended up in America, where he had what they call a cardiac ablation, which involves inserting a wire in through the groin and into the heart to basically fry the abnormal area of muscle in order to stop it producing the abnormal heart rhythm. He was cleared to return to play.

I consulted Professor Pedro Brugada, one of most eminent sports cardiologists in the world. He tested Fadiga thoroughly and we were all happy that he was fit to play. However, Brugada briefed me on what to do in the unlikely event of something untoward happening.

We took him on, everything was fine and then one cold night in October at the Reebok, the players were warming up, about to face Spurs in a league cup tie, when a coach rushed over 'Doc! Fadiga's collapsed.'

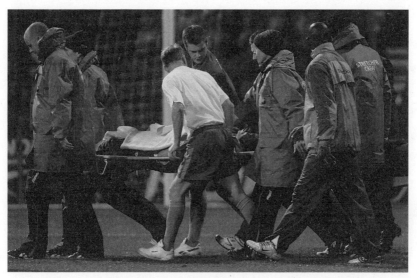

Khalilou Fadiga being carried off after collapsing in the warm-up,
BWFC v Spurs, Carling Cup tie 2004.

I dashed out to him, and there he was, unconscious on the pitch. He did have a cardiac output, but even so, this was a worst-case scenario.

'It won't happen,' Brugada had assured me, adding, 'but if it does, be prepared to act.'

Fadiga regained consciousness, was loaded onto a stretcher, taken to the medical room and hooked up to the ECG machine.

He was in what's called ventricular tachycardia, (VT) which isn't a fatal rhythm, but can soon trip into ventricular fibrillation, which is fatal unless the patient is defibrillated. VF means that basically, the heart is beating at about five hundred beats a minute but only partially filling.

The cardiac output is not able to maintain heart beat conduction and heart muscle function. The patient will usually die within a few minutes unless somebody successfully applies an electric charge to their chest, defibrillating them. Sure enough, Fadiga was going in and out of what's called VT syncope – drifting in and out of consciousness,

Usually, when you're using a defibrillator, you routinely apply 300 joules to an unconscious patient, but Professor Brugada had suggested a defibrillation charge of 30 joules. Don't wait till the heart is fibrillating, he told me, the outcome won't be as good.

It was unheard of in an adult. Maybe for a child you'd go down to thirty joules, but for an adult?

When he told me I'd just nodded, having been comforted by his previous statement that it wasn't going to happen. Now that I was here, in the medical room, having to depend on his advice to use 30 joules – *just thirty joules* . . .

But I had to put my faith in the expert.

Fortunately, this was a fully manual defibrillator from the ambulance service so I did as advised and applied a 30-joule shock to his chest.

Defibrillator charging. Fadiga looked at me. He was conscious. I tried not to think of defibrillating a conscious patient

'Stand clear!'

(Really? I was still thinking right. *Just thirty joules? And a conscious patient.)*

'Shocking!'

I delivered the charge, waited, praying for what is known as the sinus rhythm.

Got it. He reverted to normal rhythm, and thereafter remained fully consciousness – he even managed a flash of his trademark smile – and we went straight to the local coronary care unit where we spent the night.

The next day, we flew out to Belgium where he was admitted under the care of Professor Brugada and his surgical team so that they could fit an implantable defibrillator, the idea being that if and when he next developed a ventricular tachycardia, it would defibrillate him automatically. His was implanted underneath his rib cage to protect it from impact. When he returned to football, turning out for Bolton Wanderers against Ipswich in the FA Cup, he was the first professional sportsman in the world to play with an implantable defibrillator.

Allardyce was concerned – very anxious about him returning to play. But you know what I'm going to say here? It came down to our old friend informed consent; the player wanted to play. He'd had the risks explained to him and he understood them.

Ultimately, all agreed that he should be allowed to train and play for Bolton. Even the club's lawyers got involved. The Senegalese Football Association, however, needed a little persuasion. I remember, he was selected to play in a friendly in Paris, which I attended. Afterwards I interrogated his defibrillator. There's a special wand you use to check whether or not it's kicked in.

Sure enough, it had. The nerves and adrenalin rush of coming on for Senegal had triggered him into ventricular tachycardia, but the internal defibrillator had discharged and had tripped him back into normal rhythm, which of course was exactly what it was supposed to do. He had played twenty minutes without a problem.

I was concerned, though, I must admit, and the Senegalese still weren't happy. So the next international, a World Cup qualifier in Dakar, Senegal, I was invited out by Jill Fadiga, his Belgian wife, as she had serious reservations about the local medical facilities.

My wife, Frankie, came with me, and it was quite an experience to be the guest of Fadiga, who was the David Beckham of Senegal at the time, his picture on all the billboards: biscuits, washing powder – you name it, he was advertising it.

The match was held in a huge open, standing-only stadium with a ring of armed soldiers facing the crowd, grounds staff keeping those on the terraces cool with fireman's hosepipes. I sat pitchside, conscious of being one of the only white people in the stadium, clutching my defibrillator, painfully aware that Fadiga's family were pinning their hopes on me.

Sure enough, twenty minutes into the game, Fadiga stepped up to take a free kick and I saw him jump a little. Of all the thousands of people in that stadium, I was probably the only person to see him do it, but that's because I was looking for it, and of course to my eyes, it seemed obvious.

His defibrillator had gone off.

I was sweating hard from the heat (oh, yes, and the nerves), clutching my defibrillator. But if his implant had gone off, then it had clearly worked. He went on to score and win the match for Senegal.

That whole episode got me involved and passionate about proactive cardiac screening of athletes' hearts, particularly to avoid sudden unexpected cardiac death in apparently fit and healthy kids, which claims twelve young lives a week in the UK. It isn't provided on the NHS. Shortly afterwards, I met with Professor Sanjay Sharma of St Mary's Hospital in Paddington, probably the premier sports cardiologist in Britain, who heads a charity called Cardiac Risk Assessment in the Young (CRY), a free service for people aged between fourteen and thirty-five that screens for potentially avoidable causes of sudden cardiac death in young people, particularly related to exercise.

The Football Association had introduced mandatory testing for this, as had the Rugby Football Union, but arriving in cycling I discovered something of a resistance.

The problem is partly that the athletic heart is more difficult to assess than a regular heart. With its increased muscle thickness from training, you tend to get results which look abnormal but are not – so-called false positives.

Of course, you can't take any chances and so you have to withdraw the athlete until you've got a second more expert opinion. Coaches don't like that, riders don't like that. And that's what had happened at British Cycling.

Anyway, it took a bit of persuasion but I got there in the end and managed to start screening my athletes with the appropriate sports cardiology experts, introducing a policy of yearly screenings for all the podium athletes. What's more, I was finally able to wangle more cash out of the management team and extend it to the Academy.

The screening involved specialists from CRY assessing the patient, firstly with a questionnaire, and then with a clinical examination of the heart sounds with a stethoscope, a twelve-lead electrocardiogram ECG, and an ultrasound examination (ECHO), which is a functional dynamic ultrasound examination of the heart as it's pumping – the blood flow, the valve opening and closing and the thickness of the muscular walls.

The result? In Italy, twenty-five years of cardiac screening in athletes has reduced sudden cardiac death of those screened by ninety per cent. Sadly, not all conditions are detected or can be cured, but we have to make a start.

Personally, I wanted to extend the screening to any rider on a British Cycling programme aged fourteen and above, but despite proposing it in-house in early 2016 it was not picked up on as preparations for Rio 2016 were key at that time.

We should talk about some of the warning signs, which would firstly be personal history or family history of any cardiac abnormalities, which you may find helpful.

During exercise undue breathlessness, blacking out, chest palpitations (although there can be some innocent explanations). If you get any of those symptoms, they are serious and must be addressed. If someone comes to me and says that they collapsed whilst playing football, to me that's a potentially fatal cardiac arrhythmia until proven otherwise.

*　　*　　*

In January, 2017, I was devastated to hear of the sudden death of fourteen-year-old Charlie Craig, a promising British Cycling cyclo-cross programme rider, who had suffered a heart attack in his sleep.

I had never met Charlie, but even so, it had happened on my watch.

Would it have saved him if we had introduced mandatory screening, just as I wanted to in 2016? I don't know.

Immediately after his death I went to management, knowing that it was time to act. But I was told that the problems caused by Jiffygate meant that funding of the WCPP was under threat. I should get on and do my job with the podium riders.

My reaction was incredulity. And I was so concerned that I was even considering resignation, when in February 2017 I was suspended by British Cycling, for failure to keep adequate medical records, for my medicines management and for treating members of staff.

In the meantime, British Cycling appointed another head of medicine – my job – and so in September 2017, I resigned on grounds of unfair constructive dismissal.

I read the comments of the Stockport coroner Chris Morris in the press in February 2018, who said, 'It is of residual concern that British Cycling still does not routinely undertake medical evaluation or screening prior to accepting riders on to their junior training programmes.' He accepted that this may not have changed Charlie's fate, but added, 'all sports have a role to play in reducing the number of young deaths.'

I am profoundly sorry to have failed Mr and Mrs Craig's son

Charlie in not pushing harder to introduce cardiac screening for all of our athletes on all our programmes – the one time in my career that I broke my own code of protecting athletes at all costs.

I hope to use the platform of this book – as well as any other means – to raise awareness of sudden cardiac death, and help to ensure that everyone has at least one cardiac screen between the ages of fourteen and twenty. If this is you, or someone you know, go on to the CRY website and do it now.

I never screened my four kids, yet took them most Saturdays to football. I'll make sure my grandkids are screened.

Meanwhile, CPR buys time and saves lives. So get trained. Save a life. Better still, train and fundraise the purchase of your team's defibrillator. Personally, I think all professional sports should give their athletes this provision, funding the training of their staff – not just the docs and physios, but the coaches, too – and, crucially, funding for a defibrillator that's available at every training session, because the fact is, cardiac arrest and sudden cardiac death can happen anywhere, to anyone. And every athlete is somebody's kid.

If you take one thing from this book, I hope it's that.

19

If the Bike Fits . . .

*How our research at British Cycling can help you adapt your
bike to fit your body and riding style*

KEEN AMATEUR CYCLISTS SPEND a lot of money on hi-tech
bikes, which is great, but you've got to remember that there's no
point buying an expensive bike if it isn't set up properly. I see
them around and think, *That's a bad position. You'll get knee or
back pain.* If you've spent a lot of money on a bike why not
consider spending a bit more, and having a professional bike fit.

And what is one of those, you ask?

Well, it's fair to say that a lot of what's been discussed so far
has been reactive sports medicine – managing those complaints
common to cyclists, essentially firefighting; those are things that
any competent doctor would have dealt with. Where I think we
made the greatest strides at Team Sky and in British Cycling was
in creating those marginal gains I talked about – and being

proactive about the advances we made in bike fits was a great example of that philosophy in action.

At its simplest, a bike fit is making sure that the rider and bike are matched. When I first started, there was a very experienced Australian ex-rider turned coach, who used to do his bike fitting by looking out of the car as he drove past his riders and saying, 'Strewth, move it up! Move your saddle up!'

But every change creates another change somewhere else in the body. This coach had experience and intuition but the process was totally unscientific and against everything that we came to stand for at Team Sky. With this in mind, Phil Burt and I began a process whereby we'd fully assess riding position in a controlled environment using three-dimensional motion capture.

We did this by using a turbo trainer to capture rider data such as the range of movement of the leg in pedalling, especially knee extension (straightening the leg), the position of the lower back, the reach-forward and elbow position. We also captured bike data, crucially the exact height and position of the saddle.

The aim of bike fitting for the professional cyclist is to maximise power production and minimise aerodynamic drag. At the same time, we also hoped to risk-manage positions we knew were likely to produce overuse injuries, taking into account the individual's body vulnerabilities and injury history. Most bike riders, amateurs and pros, will get anterior knee pain at some time. Just think about a typical Tour stage: 90 pedal revolutions a minute, 30,000 a day. Plenty of time for an overuse injury to develop.

Our bike fit took place in a room called Room X at the

Manchester velodrome, which had restricted access and was supervised by a very bright biomechanics expert called Paul Barratt. I simply called him 'Q' for obvious reasons.

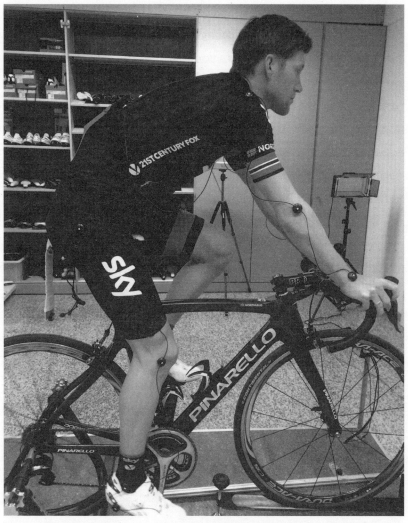

Lars Petter Nordhaug undergoing a computerised bike fit in Room X
at the Manchester Velodrome.

Most of the power in cycling comes from the gluteal muscles (the buttocks) and the quadriceps at the front of the thigh. The calf muscles are needed to transfer this power to the pedals. The iliopsoas muscle deep in the groin contributes very little, maybe more in sprinting, but is forced to operate in a crunched-up shortened position and gets tight, producing more discomfort than performance. This muscle was always a happy hunting ground for attention by the physio. As mentioned, professionals have a greater angle of knee extension for maximal power production (i.e. the leg is straighter when the pedal is at the six o'clock position.) This requires excellent hamstring and iliotibial band flexibility, and importantly allows them to roll their pelvis forward on the saddle allowing the handlebars to go low in search of aerodynamic gains.

The bike fit helped the rider achieve what is needed for performance, but also contributed to injury prevention. It could be used to great effect in injury rehabilitation where the rider might not be able to produce optimal power production or achieve a perfect aerodynamic position but could obtain a safe position to allow them to continue riding during rehab.

A surprisingly common finding I discovered is that the riders' legs were very rarely of equal length. If the difference is less than 0.5cm then most bodies can adapt. If a rider presented with a one-sided symptom, particularly pain in the sacroiliac joint, where the hip joins the pelvis, it was time for a CT scannogram of both legs, expensive but accurate to the millimetre. Rarely was it more than one cm difference and easily solved with a simple shim under the cleat on the rider's shoe.

Of course all this individual information was stored so that if a rider crashed heavily, usually meaning the carbon frame was trashed, the mechanic could replicate his exact bike set up for him. Mechanics can do a frame swap in thirty minutes, build a bike from scratch in an hour and a half. The team would get through many frames during the Tour.

The riders' spare bikes would be carried on the race car's roof rack, where there was room for nine bikes. The GC's would always be the most accessible, but swapping bikes didn't always go to plan. Occasionally, the rider would get the wrong bike, as happened to Geraint Thomas that time when he rode half a stage without noticing. Others – those 'microadjusters' – would be straight on the radio. Some riders are so sensitive to their position that they can complain their bike is not right yet often simply detecting a new saddle not yet compressed.

I'd advise any keen amateur to get a bike fit. The benefit is to prevent injury, but it will also improve rider comfort and you may even see aerodynamic gains. However, if you don't want to go the whole hog and have a professional bike fit there are certain measures you can take 'at home' as it were.

Firstly, try to ensure that when the pedal is at the three o'clock position, the front of your knee, ball of the foot and the pedal spindle are in a straight vertical line.

Next, make sure the saddle height is such that your knee is bent to about 140 degrees (i.e. with a slight bend) when the pedal is at the six o'clock position, that you have comfortable lower back position that you are capable of maintaining, as well as slightly bent elbows. This is a safe start, gradually you may be able and wish to start raising the saddle height to produce more power and go lower at the front for aerodynamic gains. Professionals have a much higher saddle position with a much straighter leg (155 degrees) at the six o'clock pedal position.

Something that is in vogue in most sports at the moment is kinesiology taping, mentioned earlier. It was a big deal to the riders at Team Sky; the tape was in Team Sky colours. But I'm not knocking that, because after all, treatment is multifactorial and is all down to a summation of marginal gains, whether it's the two litres of pineapple juice and water you take on the way to the race, your kinesiology tape, or your pre-start good-luck ritual. It all plays its part.

The biomechanics expert, Paul Barratt, was rumoured to be a member of the so-called 'Secret Squirrel Club' at British Cycling, the mystical organisation that looked for 'technical marginal gains' in each Olympic cycle.

The Secret Squirrel Club was tasked with finding as many aerodynamic tweaks as was possible within the law. A lot of time was spent in the wind tunnel, and there was a lot of work on skin suits. Eighty per cent of a rider's effort is expended in overcoming aerodynamic drag. Eighty per cent is due to the rider, twenty per cent due to the bike, and the Secret Squirrel club worked on both.

Riding on the wheel of the rider in front – i.e. sitting behind them, making the most of their draft – reduces this by 30 per cent, hence the reality that road racing is a team sport. Remember the rider at the front of the peloton will be pushing out 450 watts to maintain a speed of 40km/ph, those within it maybe just 100 watts.

Chris Boardman, Olympic gold medallist, three times World Hour Record holder, Tour de France stage winner, was the wizard in charge of the club. Some say he lived in a wind tunnel. We just called him the professor.

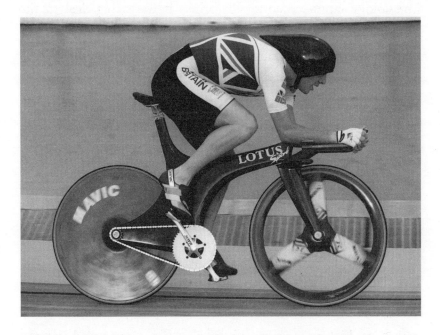

Chris Boardman MBE at Barcelona 1992, winning gold and setting the world record on the Lotus 108 bike.

This was British Cycling, something that existed before Team Sky was dreamed of. They had made some great technological advances, but it really came together for the 2012 Olympics – they were all over it, spending a lot of money on it and liaising with a lot of very bright people around the world.

20

Improving All of the Time

Training should be fun. No, wait, it should
be productive . . .

ALL TRAINING PROGRAMMES, whether for the professional or
for the committed enthusiastic amateur, should start with an
objective in mind and work backwards from there. Olympic
training plans are three years and six months long; the Tour de
France eleven months, although in truth it's continuous as each
Tour cycle builds for the next.

Coaches had differing approaches. Some would make my life
easier with a written plan (thank you, Paul Manning), others were
just a tiny a bit more tricky because they tended to store it in
their heads (Heiko Salzwedel), which could be frustrating, not
just for me, but for riders, who unsurprisingly liked to know
what the future held in store for them.

Mind you, both approaches worked: Manning and Salzwedel both coached riders to Olympic gold.

The head road gurus were Tim Kerrison, who was the Grand Tour specialist, and Rod Ellingworth, head coach at Team Sky and still men's road race coach at British Cycling from whom I learned so much, thus much of the thanks for any information here rightly goes to him.

So what is a 'training plan'? Well, in its simplest form, it's a structured programme of sufficient time, frequency and intensity to induce the bodily adaptations needed to improve aerobic and anaerobic fitness in order to achieve the desired goal.

All serious amateurs should have a plan. Some easy-to-follow ones are available to British Cycling members on their website. Ideally you need equipment to monitor your power output. You should really arm yourself with a power meter in the cranks of your pedals, as well as a GPS tracker for the handlebars, with integral data logger and software (sorry . . .). This can be uploaded to a commercial online training analysis site. It doesn't need to be expensive and accurate, as it'll be yours, so you're not comparing absolute power output with other riders, and will reference your training and hopefully demonstrate the gains you're making.

The basis of the power meter is to set your functional threshold power (FTP), which represents the maximal effort you can maintain for one hour without fatiguing. The software can calculate your normalised power which accounts for surges or spikes in power such as sprinting, closing down, climbing efforts. This is to determine how metabolically taxing the training was. Finally, it'll calculate the intensity factor – simply how intense the ride was to your threshold power.

However, while using a power meter makes things more straightforward in terms of planning, execution and analysis, than using heart-rate responses, I do think it's worthwhile wearing a chest heart-rate monitor in order to collect data. After all, the Zone 1–5 system referenced below was originally based on the increasing percentage of your maximum heart rate as you train more intensively.

How do you determine your max heart rate? Age-based calculations are often the norm, but I prefer real-time testing, either on your favourite long climb over a gradient of at least five per cent, or on a turbo trainer. To do this, first warm up on the turbo, ride at your limit for 10 minutes. And I really mean at your limit – as fast as you can go. During this, you should only be able to talk in single words; your legs should be burning. Now, unbelievably, ramp it up for another minute and then more, sprinting as fast as you can for the final 30 seconds.

This should now be producing your maximum heart rate. After warming down you can see what that figure is, providing your chest monitor hasn't malfunctioned.

Most elite riders hover just above 200bpm, but the reality is that it is largely genetically determined. Blame your parents. The higher the maximum the more potential for athletic performance you have, but it's not a sign of fitness per se. Unfortunately, it decreases with age.

You might be wondering what sort of plan the elite would follow. Pro riders train for 25 to 30 hours a week, and their diet is changed to meet the demands of their training, as well as ensuring they meet their body-fat targets. All have recovery and all have warm-up; all get reviewed and adapted; all address specific weaknesses, as well as boosting the specifics of what it takes to win, whatever type of race is the goal.

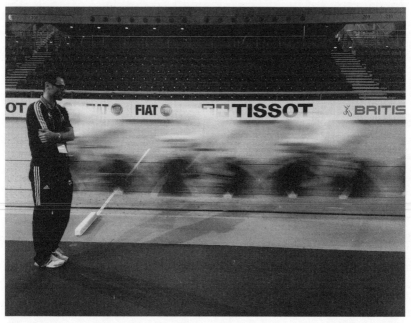

Team pursuit training by Coach Newton, Olympic track cyclist medallist, at the Lee Valley Velodrome.

So let's talk about the zone system again, which was briefly discussed in chapter 14. Training is done at different intensities to train the different energy-producing systems. Each cycling discipline has different requirements for energy. The zone systems let you train in five different zones. Each zone has a different adaptation response. They are:

Zone 1
Max heart rate: 60–65%
Percentage of rider's FTP: 56–75%
System trained: Recovery, general health maintenance
Length of ride: 1–2 hours
How does it feel? Like an easy long recovery ride.

This is an easy zone. It should feel like you're warming up as your muscles loosen and your body temperature rises. You'd use this zone to bookend more intensive zones, or if your level of fitness was low, then to build up to bigger zones. Don't neglect this zone. Don't think of it as 'lightweight'. It's very important for warming up, cooling down and recovery.

Zone 2
Max heart rate: 65–75 %
Percentage of rider's FTP: 76–90%
System trained: Aerobic energy system boosting your VO2 max to your genetic potential
Length of ride: 3–4 hour efforts
How does it feel? Like a basic training ride.

Again, a relatively light zone, but increasing in volume. It takes effort but you should be able to talk in full sentences. Imagine you're riding in a weekend bunch on the flat. You should be thinking about combining this zone with other brief but more intensive zones. But again it's a question of what suits you as an individual. What I can say is that as your fitness increases you will continue to spend time in this zone, but with increasingly longer bursts in higher zones with shorter periods of recovery at this power between them.

Zone 3

Max heart rate: 75–82%

Percentage of rider's FTP: 91–105%

System trained: Aerobic and anaerobic energy systems

System trained: Efforts of 10–30 minutes

How does it feel? Like a high-tempo ride, feeling fatigue in the legs and able to speak a few words at a time.

A beginner may only manage three minutes at this power but will soon build up with increased training. The body is mostly working just below threshold. Zone 3 is the zone that wins time trials.

Zone 4

Max heart rate: 82–89%

Percentage of rider's FTP: 106–120%

System trained: Lactic acid removal systems

System trained: Efforts of 2–10 minutes

How does it feel? Just over sustainable max power, the threshold power, legs burning. Able to speak. Only. In. Single. Words.

Training harder, the oxygen supply to the muscle runs out, and the anaerobic energy system is in command. These efforts are also known as 'spikes' and with training can be repeated with less recovery time at the lower power zone 3 between them (known as under/over training).

Zone 5

Max heart rate: 89–max heart rate

Percentage of rider's FTP: 121%+

System trained: The limited adenosine triphosphate–phospho-creatine (ATP–PC) energy system

Length of ride: Sprinting flat out, less than 2 minutes

How does it feel? Reaching VO2 max (and please see chapter 5 if you missed the bit about VO2 max), your heart and lungs are not getting enough oxygen for your muscles to produce energy. You can just grunt.

This zone is for sprinting and emptying the tank at the finish. You won't be building too much of this into your training, but you should be aiming for short bursts as your condition improves. You'll know when you're ready for it.

How does that all work in practice? I have myself as an example, because I'm planning to race my first 10km time trial soon. This is a sensible distance to train for, as it avoids the risks of the peloton and man-on-man racing with a rival. I'm aiming for a 24-minute time, and I reckon I can spend 12 hours per week training.

To do it, I have a turbo trainer in the garage so I can be certain of some quality training whatever the weather. My coach (Paul Manning) has planned three-hour-long endurance rides in Zone 2, as well as other rides with spikes into Zones 3 and maybe briefly into 4. The former – Zone 3 – is the sustained power I'm aiming to race, and so I'll be doing three-minute spikes into that zone.

As the weeks progress, Manning has planned more volume with less rest between efforts, soon I'll be doing 4 x 6 minutes Zone 3 efforts with easy riding between them, working through

2 x 12 minute efforts. Finally, the week before the time trial I'll do a race rehearsal: a full 24 minutes at my threshold power output.

Then I'll back off, taper and allow the adaptions of training to occur and enough recovery to get super-compensation.

Coach Manning has advised me not to go off too fast. His advice is to stay in Zone 3, don't spike into Zone 4 and blow (i.e. be overwhelmed by lactic acid). This is especially important in the race, with the adrenalin pumping, and I've seen it happen to many elite riders in the heat of battle. Zone 4 is for gradients and unexpected head winds.

As for posture, Coach Manning recommends a low flat back minimising my frontal area but urges me to choose a position I can hold, that doesn't put me at risk of injury and allows me to produce my power. And to practise holding a good position in training ready for racing

My helmet is a short one, made by KASK, as I'm prone to bobbing about with my head and need to see where I'm going. The very long tapered aero helmets don't allow much movement of the head, are hard to see out of and easily steam up.

Of course I won't forget to build in recovery periods. Nobody should. All training effects need time for the adaptions to appear and give the planned-for super-compensation. So a weekly plan should be skewed – starting heavily, carrying fatigue into the later lighter training and then recovery. We'll talk about recovery in greater detail in the next chapter.

As always a healthy balanced diet is key, as is staying fuelled and hydrated on the bike, as well as consuming recovery protein and carbs within that vital 'golden hour' of finishing the session apply to all. Good-quality sleep is also essential. Illness and injury – not to mention family activities – may mean the plan has to be adapted, so bear that in mind.

Cross training, say swimming or conditioning in the gym, should all be factored in as well as pressure-point foam rolling in the glutes and stretching afterwards, especially the iliotibial band (please go online to familiarise yourself with this fascia – more on fascia later), gluteals and quadriceps. If it's affordable, splash out on a weekly soft-tissue massage on recovery days. You might even think about treating yourself by refuelling with – you've guessed it – chocolate milk.

21

Recovery

It's as important as training, but often neglected –
this is how best to let your body make the most
of its downtime . . .

'OVER-TRAINING SYNDROME' was a condition first noted by
the Medical and Scientific Director of the International Olympic
Committee, Richard Budgett.

Dr Budgett was an Olympic rower and a doctor who subsequently became the Medical Director of the British Olympic
Association, and he had identified this condition suffered by
elite athletes, whereby an athlete with a high training volume
or abruptly increasing training volume starts to perform badly
in training or in races; as a result of which they immediately
think, *Damn, I'm not training enough*, and decide to solve the
problem by training more, which in turn makes the situation
worse.

That's over-training syndrome, which if unchecked can ultimately lead to immune function breakdown, hormonal dysfunction, mental ill-health and increased risk of injury.

The essence of training is a progressive overload to the body's physiology, stimulating adaptation, leading to an increase in performance. Riders train to win races. The more the training load reproduces their specific sport's stress, the more races they'll win.

In cycling, the coaches use many strategies to increase physiological stress within training: riders may go to train at altitude up a mountain or in a hypoxic chamber (in which the oxygen in the air is reduced). They may even sleep in a hypoxic tent. Some train in an environmental chamber with increased humidity and temperature in order to replicate the conditions they'll be competing in, the idea being to increase sustained power output for racing, time trialling and climbing, and anaerobic bursts for surges and sprinting – whatever the environmental conditions. All of which win races.

This was a training remit brought into cycling by Brailsford. A brave new world of training where simply logging six-hour bike rides became a thing of the past. Instead riders worked specifically on the task at hand, training in the same climbs or gradients they would face in the upcoming Tour de France, for example.

As a result, however, they were constantly at risk of over-training.

When I came into cycling I saw that the coaches were driving athletes to the edge. Some were good and pulled back before they broke the riders, but others would just push, and push and so it was the doctor's role then to say, 'Whoa, just stop, you're over-training them, we need some more recovery.' Sometimes it's psychological recovery, not just physical. Either way, this assessment that 'enough is enough' is the essential skill of a sports doctor, because when an athlete breaks, it's never the coaches' fault, nor the athlete's. The finger points towards the doctor and the medical and sport science support team. Wayne Rooney's stress fracture, an overload fracture, didn't lead to either him or the manager leaving the club. No, the doctor left.

But of course I also knew – another of my many mantras – that all professional sport is unhealthy. I knew that riders will often train or compete when they're ill or injured. The trick is working out to what degree an athlete or coach is prepared to do it. Some train when they've got massive injury problems and their pain thresholds are immense. Others will pull out sooner.

Moreover, some athletes can carry this overload, this feeling of fatigue, whilst continuing training and not break down, and this sets them apart as possessing optimal trainability. They're the same athletes that you rarely see in the medical room, who know their own bodies and have the confidence to inform their coach.

I looked at the training that these riders were doing, and turned this equation on its head. To me this was not a question of over-training. The problem was under-recovery – and it was that I should be monitoring. That philosophy became one of the bedrocks of the way that I helped athletes, by ensuring they had enough recovery, either by negotiating reduced training load or more rest days.

First job. To find some way of monitoring the athletes. To this end, and with the help of colleagues at the English Institute of Sport, we introduced a phone app to help monitor recovery, which the riders were asked to complete and upload each morning on waking:

How well did you sleep?
How long did you sleep?
What was your average sleeping heart rate? (measured by a Fitbit watch)
Do you feel tired?
Do you have excessive muscle soreness?
What was your perceived effort of exertion for yesterday's session?
Did you complete the session?
What is your mood?

As a snapshot it was pretty useless data. But day by day, week by week, what we term longitudinal data was produced and this showed the rider's normal responses and trends. It became invaluable for detecting subtle changes away from the individual's norm.

The men's team pursuit went one step further. Each morning they'd do a ramp test on their turbo trainers, riding at three increasing intensities and recording their heart rate response at each intensity and the rate of its recovery in the warm-down.

A heart rate too high or a slow return to normal all suggested under-recovery and overload of stress on the body.

This was the gold-standard test for cyclists, but what I'd

recommend for the amateur is the questions and a Fitbit watch – or just the watch.

Either way, you need time off for recovery, and while we can try to be clever in medicine it's usually just a case of allowing the body time to adapt or even heal. David Beckham needed a certain length of time for that metatarsal to heal. They may have tried special ultrasound wave treatments; they might have tried hyperbaric oxygen chambers. But essentially you're observing a biological process evolved over thousands of years, and it's unmoved by the match you have next Saturday.

So how did this recovery theory work in action, on a day-to-day basis? How can you make it work for you?

Once you get into the race season, riders are lucky to have a good day's recovery after they finish a race. It's vital to have, but it's not absolute recovery. Athletes are like racehorses, they need to exercise daily and they need to run, so I would never suggest a rider did nothing on their recovery days, just a light spin, maybe, two to four hours, which sounds a lot but it's not exertion for them so they're not getting a training effect, they're just mobilising the muscles, the joints, stressing the heart, the lungs and getting the blood that's needed for healing circulating to their damaged tissues. They need that for their legs as well as the soft-tissue massage on a daily basis, which is so important for the muscles.

The main means of recovery in cycling is 'active rest' and time away from exertion. Recovery and expending as little energy as possible go hand in hand, which for cyclists means walking about as little as possible. This doesn't mean no activity at all though.

The Line

At the Olympics in 2012 and 2016 we supplied each rider with a bike, a little runaround so they could ride to media commitments, to the food hall or to meet their family and friends outside.

Now, you might say that by cycling they were also using precious energy and of course you'd be partly right, but cyclists are cyclists and they use those muscles; a cyclist will prefer to jump on a bike and cycle to the toilet at the track rather than put on trainers and walk there. Are you conserving energy? Are you imprinting that cycling action on your muscles? Marginal gains? I don't think there's an answer to that. I do know that it was something that they themselves instigated and what a rider wants a rider usually gets.

In the meantime, recovery begins right away after an event, and it needs to be planned. Some events are sequential; there may be two or more rides on the same day or a final round and then a final, and of course if that's the case then the approach needs to be tailored accordingly, but if we're talking about a standard event, then recovery starts immediately: riders get their media and whatever else they need to do out of the way as soon as possible then work on taking their protein replacement as quickly as they can and getting back to their accommodation as fast as possible. They're advised to wear compression tights on the lower limbs, though whether they follow that advice often comes down to whether they can stand that pressure on overheated, sore, tired muscles. There's no doubting that it's good for the muscles and helps reduce tissue swelling, it's just that some athletes can't take it.

The compression garments we used at Team Sky were bespoke, but your own tape measure and a reputable supplier with sizing by average measurement is more than adequate.

Recovery

Meanwhile, once back at the hotel, everybody would rest. Heard the one about the athlete sitting in a hotel lobby after an event? No, because it would never happen. They're either resting, having treatment with the soft-tissue therapist, or the physiotherapist, or being seen, assessed and tended to by the doctor, or – and this very common indeed for stage riders – flat on their backs in bed with their legs elevated. Stretches, soft-tissue rolling and pressure-point work can be done before bed or the next day.

They'd begin rehydrating right away. We recommended getting rehydration started as early as possible in order to prevent riders having to get up at 2am and disturb their sleep for a pee.

Recovery happens when you're resting, but recovery really happens when you're asleep. It's poorly understood, but hormones are released when you're asleep, very important hormones for a healthy body. The earlier I could get the riders to lights out, and the later I could get the riders to lie in and potentially sleep for longer, the better; some days, we had a golden opportunity where we could have a later start, because our hotel was close to the next stage start or the riders had a later event at the track. So, sleep, sleep, sleep – more on which later.

Other means of recovery? You may have heard of intravenous recovery, which is sticking a needle into an athlete and injecting him or her with nutrients.

It had been a common practice in cycling. However, I didn't believe in it, and thought it was simply a case of the placebo effect. Any conflict that might have flared up between my approach and that of the old school was headed off at the pass, when in May 2011, the 'no needles' policy was introduced into cycling (by the UCI doctor, Mario Zorzoli) meaning that no injections were allowed when racing.

Anyway, Nigel Mitchell, the nutritionist, had always believed we could provide what was required orally, and together we worked hard to make sure we could, and to concentrate on having them eat 'proper' food, a super healthy diet as it was to be known. With that in mind, we had open access to food rooms at BC and Team Sky, where all the appropriate recovery nutrition was on offer, whether that was natural health products, ranging from nuts to dried fruit, cereal, full-fat milk and yoghurt or protein bars – horrible-tasting things, like chewing a mixture of cardboard and rubber, normally flavoured with orange – and of course protein powder. Riders would often take a scoop at bedtime. We also used sequential pneumatic compression boots and trousers, which squeezed from the feet to the groin, attempting to 'milk' the swelling in the fatigued lower legs back to the circulation.

Another form of recovery is ice-based recovery. Something we found essential when injury was involved was the ice-compression cuff. There's a variety of sizes of cuffs suitable for all the injured parts. Wrist cuff, knee cuff, and so on.

The cuffs were fitted then ice-cold water was pumped in to compress and cool the area. We had half a dozen of them and they travelled the world with us. This device is literally a game-changer in acute injury management. You can get them online or at sports shops – from expensive contraptions similar to the ones we used, right down to gel packs and compression cuffs for just over a fiver.

Something we tried at Bolton was whole-body cryotherapy,

which was essentially a sauna in reverse. Athletes walked in and were subjected to a physiological shock of dry absolutely freezing-cold air.

Most operate at minus 120 degrees Celsius. The one we had at Bolton when we were shaking it down reached minus 192, possibly the coldest place in Britain that day.

You can get portable chambers that are run on liquid nitrogen, and they're increasingly popular in football and rugby – premierships, usually, as it's an expensive treatment. Players wear just briefs for maximal skin exposure, and gloves, trainers and a headband to prevent their extremities getting frostnip (although technically that shouldn't happen, because it's a moisture-free atmosphere). The effect was that feeling of '*Ahhhhh!*' – two minutes of extreme cold shock followed by sensations of exquisite pleasure when users escape back out into the warmth.

Are we back with the placebo effect again? Does it work? Does it *really* work, except in the minds of those using it? And is there a difference?

I firmly believe it does have a recovery effect, especially in contact sport, for reasons yet to be proven. Personally, I loved it and would use it on a daily basis once the players had been processed. As for the players, there were some who opposed it, but then there was a certain type of player who opposed everything – didn't like being advised on recovery, on what to eat, on when to wear compression tights, anything. You didn't get that kind of resistance so much in cycling. In football we had to rely on getting a key dressing-room leader on board, which during my time with Wanderers was Speed.

The Line

Prior to the cryotherapy chamber we used ice baths.

We tend to lump them together, ice baths and whole-body cryotherapy, but they do quite different things, in my opinion. The ice bath certainly has a muscle-cooling effect, and will help to limit swelling from tissue damage, which is especially applicable to contact sports; where there's more contact, there's more bruising and microscopic haemorrhage. Cryotherapy was much more of a systemic shock, and suitable for all sports. However, both help the subjective feeling of recovery.

In the treatment room you need a machine that produces ice, lots of it, which is common in professional sport because of course you need ice all the time. Ice is an essential part of sports medicine. Why? Because the four mainstays of treatment of an injury are RICE: rest, ice, compression, elevation. An acute injury, you obviously diagnose it first, then you rest it, you ice it – cooling helps stop bleeding and tissue fluid production – you compress it – strap an ankle up that's strained for instance – and then you elevate it, all the while trying to limit swelling which can slow down recovery.

So you have machines that make different forms of ice. Some make a slushy ice, which is great, because that just goes in a bag and it's already melted and it's easy to mould around the injured part. Some make ice cubes, which are good for ice baths.

You probably don't have a machine at home, so either invest in an ice pack that you keep in the fridge or remember the bag of frozen peas: apply to the injured area three repetitions of two minutes on, two minutes off. Remember to avoid ice burns, so cover the injury with a wet tea towel first.

So I came to Team Sky with all this thinking under my belt, the whining of the players still ringing in my ears; that space-age cryotherapy chamber was still fresh in my mind (it fell into disuse after Allardyce left – I think they used it as a store cupboard) and I wanted to bring all of this recovery thinking to the riders. The main man – the GC contender – at the time was Wiggins, and he was willing to give it a try. Well, that was different to football for a start. Cycling, they're hard men; football, they're, well, more 'sensitive'.

So we bought ourselves an inflatable ice bath, trialled it and then lugged it around France for three weeks. It was difficult. We had to have someone go ahead and inflate the ice bath, which was too big for the average hotel bathroom and would usually have to go in a corridor or sometimes in my bedroom. Then the poor old swannies would have to fill it, having pre-warned the hotel to order six sacks of ice.

Any riders who had active bleeding were excluded from using it, but invariably it was only Wiggins who went in anyway, bleeding or not, and in fact there's a great picture of him using it in his book, looking resigned, while sporting the typically gaunt Tour de France look.

Then the ice bath would have to be drained, which was difficult, seeing that it was either in a corridor or next to my bed, and then it had to be cleaned with antiseptic.

As you might imagine, the ice bath didn't last long. Instead we stuck to the basic tenets: rest, compression massage, compression tights, sleep.

Talking of which . . .

22

The Reason That French Hotels Groaned When We Showed Up

The benefits of sleep hygiene and associated marginal gains

WHEN TRAVELLING, WE WOULD PROVIDE riders with a travel pack. This was specific to Team Sky. With British Cycling we'd all travel together, en masse, so everything would come with us, whereas our Sky riders arrived from all over the world and thus were issued with this travel pack I put together.

In it would be hand sanitiser, oral zinc lozenges and zinc nasal spray.

British Cycling *would* get their own travel packs if we were on long-haul flights. This would also include easy-to-eat nutritious foods, such as plenty of dried fruit and nuts, yoghurt, protein bars and Pot Noodles, because some of the food provided by planes in economy class, which we invariably flew, was either nutritionally poor or of insufficient quantity to meet the riders' calorie requirements.

Infection control is also a big issue when travelling, especially flying because the air we breathe is re-circulated many times. We made sure that riders weren't seated next to a spluttering, coughing member of the public, if necessary acting as buffers ourselves. At the same time, all riders would have zinc lozenges to suck and zinc nasal spray to use. Zinc has a potent effect on viral infection in the throat and nose, and planes are a potent source of viral infections. It's always a good idea to take zinc when you travel.

When we were really turning the heat up for the World Championships in Melbourne before the Olympics in 2012, we decided that flying business class was an uncontroversial but expensive marginal gain, so the riders – but not the staff – should fly in bed in order that they could rest and sleep better. The only time I almost got to turn left on a flight was when the call came: if there's a doctor on board please inform the cabin crew. It was something I'd done many times before, helping someone in trouble with skills I'd been given. I hoped that if it came to it, another doctor would do the same for my family. Besides I enjoyed the responsibility and the challenge.

There's a lot of science about how to acclimatise to changing time zones. People have tried tricking themselves by changing watches, using night lights, going to bed early when you arrive, keeping the curtains open later – all sorts of things which no doubt have some benefit.

However, the best way to acclimatise quickly when you travel across time zones is to put sleep in the sleep bank, simple as that. So, as soon as you got on that plane, eat, drink, no alcohol, and fall asleep. It was one of the few occasions when I let them have a sleeping tablet. For that same reason we tried to time flights so that they were in the middle of the day, to avoid the need for those shattering early starts that can take days to recover from. Straightforward travel fatigue.

All of which brings me on to 'sleep hygiene', one of our key marginal gains.

I'm pleased to say that the world at large is finally coming around to the enormous health benefits of a good night's sleep, but we at Team Sky were well ahead of the game in that respect. Dr Peters was very keen on sleep as a mental health recovery strategy and had experience of the behavioural management of it, rather than drug management (prescribing sleeping tablets), which was an unusual approach at the time. He knew that although sleep hygiene was as important for the man in the street as it was for the professional athlete, there are certain reasons why professional athletes – particularly elite cyclists – have trouble sleeping.

Firstly, there's all that blasted caffeine I've been railing against. Coffee in the morning followed by caffeine gels throughout the day. That's an awful lot of mental stimulation. Also, you're asking a lot of the body to metabolise it in time for bed.

Of course, I would have preferred a simple 'no caffeine' rule. But hey, you choose your battles and that was one I could never win, particularly with the cycling coffee culture as it was. What's more I was still a great believer in informed consent and patient autonomy. I could tell a rider why I thought it was a good idea to decrease, even cut out caffeine entirely till race day, but I couldn't force them.

'I'll have another double espresso, Doc, do you want one?'

'Yeah, all right, then.'

I was a green tea drinker at Bolton, I was a double espresso drinker on the Death Star. Says it all.

However, I did get most of the riders to restrict their intake or at least acknowledge that they were taking too much, which I believe led to better behaviour in future.

It's exactly the same with sleeping tablets. When I arrived at Team Sky one of the many major surprises was the huge demand for sleeping tablets from the riders. Some even had their own suppliers, not necessarily doctors.

At British Cycling they were used infrequently, and that tended to be when we were on long-haul flights or were changing time zones, but at Team Sky there was a different attitude; it was almost routine. They were stimulated by caffeine – all day, throughout the day – and then took a tablet to get them to sleep at night.

It was crazy. *Stimulant. Sleep. Stimulant. Sleep*. The problem being that when you use sleeping tablets, the quality of sleep, that so-called REM, or Rapid Eye Movement sleep – is compromised, so although you're asleep, which is better than lying there staring at the ceiling, you're not in that repairing, restorative phase of sleep.

It was no different to my days in general practice. The general population will sleep badly for a variety of reasons: problems at work, problems with relationships, kids, worry, anxiety, stress, mobile phones, laptops, TVs in the bedroom – all reasons you'd recognise. And most of them want a pill. Sleeping tablets have their place, for short-term use, to get back into a healthy sleeping pattern, but not long-term maintenance as it leads to dependency and increased tolerance and therefore the need to increase the dose. For some it can lead to addiction and abuse.

There's an expert in everything, so we got one in. At Bolton, we'd bought a number of top-quality memory foam mattresses and set them up at the training ground in order for players to rest between training sessions. It wasn't unknown for us to simply buy one of these mattresses for a player to have at home if we thought it would help. Again, lots of support from the ever-progressive Allardyce for that particular innovation.

So we asked a sleep consultant to visit the velodrome, and he arrived with lots of theory and advice, and plenty of sample mattresses, pillows, and duvets that he left behind for athletes to try at home, the simple reason being that people sleep better in their own beds. You might know yourself that if you spend one night in a hotel, you tend to sleep poorly, but if you stay a second night you then sleep better.

For our riders, especially Team Sky, this presented a particular problem, because they were changing hotels every night.

The idea, then, was that they should take their bedding with them on tour. Each rider selected what he was most comfortable with. Some liked thick, warm duvets, some liked thinner ones. It was the same with mattress and pillow firmness. Needless to say, the duvets, pillows, mattresses and the bed linen were all hypo-allergenic.

We dedicated a van and driver to the task of carting that lot around France everywhere we went. A pretty big task. We'd roll up at a hotel, take all the mattresses out of the rooms, and then bring our own in.

Not only that, but we'd have the support staff hoover the rooms in order to get rid of pollen and dust and especially house dust mites that feed on skin flakes from the previous guest. A lot of children wheeze or cough at night and often that's because of the huge allergy load in a bedroom from the carpet and mattress which are full of these house dust mites feeding on the skin flakes. Support staff would hoover the room, hoover the mattresses, damp dust everywhere – do all they could to make sure that the room wasn't just clean, but deep clean.

Laundry – that was something else that bothered us. The bigger hotels would have their laundry done in the basement but we'd arrive at a lovely quiet French village-type hotel and see linen on lines outside, floating in the breeze. The skies were blue, the sun was warm, you were in a beautiful part of France and it felt wonderful.

Downside? Those sheets and pillowcases were picking up pollen so when they were brought in and put on the beds, they were allergen bombs. We had to stop that. No way did we want to bring a massive dose of pollen into the rooms of athletes who were already struggling with allergies from a day's racing through fields of sunflowers. I'd advise that for anyone with a child with night-time allergies (or who has one themselves): remove the carpet and don't dry your sheets outside on a lovely sunny day.

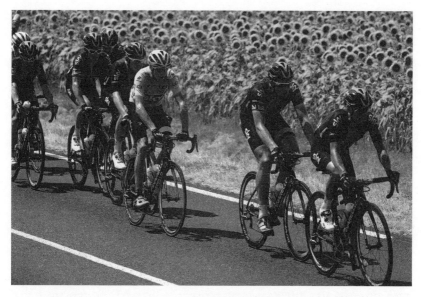

Sunflowers, stage 13, 2015 Tour de France, beautiful to look at but giving a very high pollen count.

Washing powder was something else we watched carefully, having had some riders allergic to biological types. Again, it was something we couldn't regulate at hotels so we took our own non-biological washing powder for the washing machines in the mechanics' trucks.

As you might imagine, hotels didn't exactly greet us with open arms. There was no: 'We're so honoured to have you staying here. How can we make your stay more pleasant?'

For a start, they were French hotels and we were a British team, and the French didn't like being told anything by the British, certainly not in a cycling context, because the Tour de France was the crown jewels of France. First the Americans had had the audacity to come and take the title, and then Brailsford had come along and announced that a British Team – not only that, but a British rider – was going to win it. 'Oh, la la.'

Reason two: because the Tour organisers were the ones booking and paying for the hotels, and you can bet they weren't paying top dollar. Like any other business they have to keep an eye on the purse strings. So certainly some of the food we used to get reflected that. We'll come to why this increased their dislike of us in a moment.

And thirdly, and perhaps most importantly, we were just a huge pain in the arse for them. After all, what guest arrives at a hotel and brings not only their own bedding, which they insist is washed in their own washing powder and not hung out to dry outside, but also their own mattresses? Oh, and the mattress that was in the room has to be taken away from the delicate airways of the riders and stored elsewhere in the hotel.

You could hardly blame them for being less than pleased – and that was before we even came on to the subject of food.

We did that for about a year, carting mattresses around with us. But it was too much effort, logistically. So then we moved on to mattress toppers, and riders would have their own duvet and pillow. I think having your own pillow is probably the most important.

Blackout blinds. That was another one. Some riders like it darker than dark when they're trying to sleep, and indeed that would be a great help when we were changing time zones – for example, travelling to Rio.

There was one particular rider at British Cycling for whom we got blackout blinds whether she was at the holding camp, the

Worlds or the Olympics, but even so she still slept with an eye mask on and earplugs in. She couldn't get to sleep without it all. She needed that total sensory blackout. She also insisted on rooming alone.

Similarly, we used special lights at breakfast – so-called SAD lamps (Seasonal Affective Disorder). They produce an extra-bright light. We used them at breakfast, setting them up next to the hand sanitiser. The idea is that they stimulate your pineal gland (which is where melatonin, the 'sleep hormone' that affects the wake/sleep cycle, is produced) and therefore help with adapting to time zones when travelling and energy in the winter. Next, we tried to instruct riders to limit bright screen use around bedtime. We had a rule that *at least* half an hour, but certainly preferably an hour, before bed tablets, computers or phones were put away. The simple reason being that it has now been proved that these screens disrupt your sleep because they emit blue light that disrupts the production of melatonin.

Perhaps confusingly I do not feel supplementation with oral melatonin is effective. It's as usual much more complicated than that.

Needless to say, it was difficult to get riders to cooperate with the no-screen rule, but we tried. I'd always do a 'ward round', a final sweep last thing at night, when I'd visit each of the rider's rooms to check that all was well.

I'd go into the room only to discover that they had been too exhausted to even get out of bed. The light would be off when it should be on, or the light would be on when it was supposed to be off. They'd gone from dusk to dark without the energy to do anything except look at their screens. They shared rooms and I'd go in and see two bright white screens on the bed. Not only was there the issue of light, but also the mental overstimulation involved, where they're checking Twitter and getting angry because some keyboard warrior has had a go at them.

I'd tell hotel reception that under no circumstances was a rider to be disturbed at night, no calls were to be put through. They were always to call me first. Even if doping control arrived. I made sure that the rooming list was never pinned up in the corridor for anyone passing to see, in case some fan tried to get in touch, or worse be malicious and wake somebody up.

Another thing we had to bear in mind was room temperature. Obviously it's a matter of taste, but in trials most people will sleep better if the room temperature is around 18 degrees. If you want to work out your own optimum room temperature, I'd advise starting at 18 degrees and going from there.

We decided an optimal temperature was a marginal gain and so we would use our own portable air-conditioning if it was unavailable. Some riders didn't like air conditioning, because they felt it dried the air. Which is reasonable.

On top of all that, Dr Peters would give riders a behavioural talk on sleep management at the new season's training camp. One method for getting to sleep was relax all the muscles in the body starting at your head, moving down to your toes, the idea being that within thirty seconds of not moving and doing that you'd be asleep. Cards on the table, I tried it and it never worked for me. However, behavioural forms of management really took off in British Cycling, where they'd do a relaxation class before going to bed, complete with appropriate background music and their own pillows. Personally I thought it was a superb way to prepare for sleep, and I was a great believer. Watching the class always reminded me of seeing my kids play 'sleeping lions' at day nursery.

Lastly, my secret weapon. Something I would always carry in my doctor's bag was camomile tea bags. Possibly they were an example of the placebo effect at work, but they were very effective and I used them again and again. As a helpful trick for getting to sleep, I liked it, the riders seemed to like it and it became one of those things, a bit like the Fishermen's Friends – you could always get camomile tea from the Doc.

23

A Drink That Looks Like a Stool Sample, and Other Delicacies

In order to get the best out of your body, you need to watch what you put in . . .

No DOUBT ABOUT IT, CYCLISTS put some crap into their bodies. I'll give you an example. At British Cycling, we worked closely with the University of Manchester Dental Hospital who did a lot of research into the state of our athletes' teeth.

Not surprisingly, what we discovered was that the riders' teeth were in a terrible state, mainly because of all the energy drinks they consume while training. Six hours of training, constantly glugging these syrupy drinks and never rinsing their mouths afterwards took its toll – many riders suffered with dental problems.

I thought, *There's a marginal gain here.* Their teeth could be holding them back. Because after all, there have to be deleterious effects from micro-infection. Certainly there would be with a dental abscess just before a World Championship or an Olympic Games.

So, we teamed up with the Dental School, who gave us open access to the dental hospital and its brilliant consultant-led care whenever we wanted.

Of course, that was for general dental care, but it was also for trauma, because as you can imagine, riders often damage their teeth when falling off.

But still, it's an example of how something seen as a short-term gain (e.g. an energy drink) can have long-term drawbacks, and goes back to my oft-made point about balancing the two.

It also illustrates the role played by diet in what we do.

A lot has been said about cycling and weight management. Whenever I looked after tour riders, the main issue was getting them to maintain their ideal race weight or 'target weight' that was set and agreed before they started the race.

The target weight is the ideal power-to-weight ratio for climbing over mountains. Lean muscle mass versus fat stores: that's the balance that riders must always strike. It's fair enough losing most of your subcutaneous fat – that's a performance gain – but soon enough you start to lose muscle mass. When you lose muscle mass, you lose power, and there's no point in being light and weak.

So how does this work in terms of diet? When I first arrived on the cycling scene most riders seemed to survive on a handful of supplements, together with lots of pasta. So one of the first things I did was to get them off excess pasta (wheat), which went against what was the current thinking in sport. Most people were used to the idea of footballers or marathon runners loading up on pasta before a big event. However, it's my opinion that too much wheat gives athletes a gluten intolerance as well as what I call a leaky bowel, both of which can lead to abdominal bloating. Also some riders seemed to develop a mild lactose intolerance when stressed to the limit so I'd have to be careful with milk, different to my experience at the football club and on the track.

So it was rice and chicken or chicken and rice. Too bad.

Salmon was also popular, salmon and chicken both being easy-to-digest sources of quality protein. Rice and potatoes were their carbohydrate source. Very occasionally on tour, because three weeks is a long time, they could have steak, but of course red meat takes longer to digest and the riders don't want anything extra in their gut whatsoever.

What happens during a Grand Tour is that riders easily get a negative energy balance because they simply can't keep up with calorific intake – a real war of attrition.

The Grand Tour often starts on the flat for a week, fighting and sprinting, then it heads into the high mountains and as it heads into the high mountains, the athletes make sure that their bowels are empty, because 2kg extra weight when climbing over the peak is significant.

We worked on refining that process. As we entered the mountains section of the race, riders would go on what we call 'a low residue diet', which meant cutting down on diet roughage so that their stools were less bulky. Long term it's not particularly good for your health, to be honest, but for three weeks it's okay.

After the departure of Nigel Mitchell we employed a professor of nutrition, Dr James Morton, who had previously worked with Liverpool FC.

What he brought to the team was a more scientific approach. Instead of just having a good idea, he was able to quantify it. The professor calculated how much protein/carbohydrate/fat was needed and in what form. He worked with the athletes on a one-to-one basis. He worked on instructing the *soigneurs* who prepared in-race feeding, which evolved into the professor advising what food the team (and it was 'the team', not just the riders) should have for breakfast, at training camps and races. I always encouraged a daily small bottle of probiotics with breakfast to optimise gut health.

In turn that evolved into us having our own chef working in the hotel kitchen (which was not welcomed with open arms by the resident French chefs) which then evolved into taking our own travelling kitchen/dining room on tour with us, the idea being that the athletes at Team Sky should want for nothing nutritionally. And we could completely control sources of food and ensure absolute hygiene.

Reluctantly the swannies even started to use food handlers' gloves when they prepared the in-race foods. Habits are hard to break, and to be fair we'd not had much doubt about their hand washing, they were very professional and prepared their little preparation area on the mechanics truck with care, so much so that I turned a blind eye when I often saw the box of gloves unopened. That requirement faded away, and the swannies got on with their work as before.

I enjoyed watching the daily ritual of the preparation of race food and liquid, listening to the banter ahead of the day's racing. Swannies are committed to the sport, passionate about cycling; it's a way of life, with so much time necessarily away from home. Always one more task asked from them, but not once did I see them complain.

Meanwhile, British Cycling did their best to keep up with their well-fed colleagues at Team Sky, but there were cost implications there, so while the BC riders enjoyed excellent food and nutritional management while either at training camps or at major competitions, at the velodrome they had to fend for themselves. They ate in a canteen open to the public, serving chips and cake as daily temptations, which they paid for themselves.

At home, they budgeted for buying their own healthy food and preparing it themselves. Some are very good at that and had the skills and knowledge to do it properly, some were less successful and would be tempted for pizza.

An obvious marginal gain when we were coming up into major competitions, the Worlds or Olympics, was that we'd start using in-house catering, so they ate a high-quality, nutritious meal before or especially after training, paid for by the programme. Not only was it good for them it was good for team morale – nothing better than getting all your riders sitting down together – as it has a real bonding effect.

So what should you, the amateur, be eating? Basically you have to eat the right stuff in the right proportion and there's nothing like freshly prepared food. Anything processed has unknown amounts of salt or even sugar added, so that's a complete nonstarter. Vegetables, especially leafy greens, have no limit. Smoothies made from vegetables were very popular and the riders consumed vast amounts of those.

Usually, the trouble when you prepare vegetables is that you overcook them and boil them for too long, thus you damage the very nutrients you want to get out of them.

A vegetable smoothie was an ideal way of getting around this problem. Some were absolutely delicious, some were appalling, some looked beautiful, others like a brown loose stool sample. In any case, they interrupted the nutritional boredom of a constant diet of rice and chicken.

What is important to realise is that the rider's calorific intake has to be determined by their training or racing load. They should never be hungry, and their calorific intake, whether it's protein, fat or carbohydrate, is massive. A rider needs 5,000 quality calories a day, every day, to survive a Grand Tour – about 2½ times the amount a normal person requires in any single day – and should drink around ten litres a day, which is a vast amount. So a rider is always playing catch-up, and that's where Grand Tour ambitions can start to unravel because ultimately riders can't maintain the calorific intake, have burned up all their body fat and then start catabolising lean muscle mass. Losing power.

That's catabolising, by the way, not metabolising, which is just a biological process. If something is being catabolised, it's being broken down. The reverse is anabolic, which means building up. So, an anabolic steroid will hypertrophy a muscle, in other words make it bigger, somewhat stronger. However, the quality of this change isn't as good as twenty years pushing weights; as I've said, just look at Hoy.

A typical race-day diet

The day begins with breakfast, which any athlete or sports nutritionist will tell you is the most important meal of the day. It's their opportunity to charge their energy stores for the day's exercise. Energy can be stored in various parts of the body, it can be stored in muscles, in body fat and it can be generated as glucose in the liver from a whole variety of things. That's why they always go with high protein and high carbohydrate at breakfast: scrambled eggs, yoghurt, omelette and porridge with lots of honey. Plus the obligatory coffee after which we try to get them to have their two litres of water mixed with fruit juice – pineapple juice it was in the end.

When it came to race food, it varied a lot between teams, but there was always a selection in the musette. They loved frangipane cake, some would have sandwiches, ham or jam. They would have to eat all of this on the bike, but it was specially wrapped in foil, and would be unwrapped riding no-handed. And, of course, protein bars and lots and lots of gels, which would be just carbohydrate or sometimes with added caffeine.

As previously mentioned, a very popular foodstuff for on-bike eating was a special rice cake, a Mitchell speciality, a mixture of rice, Nutella and cream cheese, which was made the night before in a rice cooker and left in the fridge overnight. By morning it was solid and cut into bite-sized portions. I loved it.

The great thing about the rice cakes, apart from the taste, was that they wouldn't melt in the riders' jersey pockets which is vital in the high temperatures experienced in racing. Anyone who uses gels, whatever their alleged flavour, agrees that something to refresh your palate is very welcome.

So they'd start the race with lots of food in their pouches in the backs of their race jerseys – not too much, that would mean too much weight to carry. After a certain mileage the race radio would announce 'the bar is open' meaning feeding and drinking from the car was allowed. The *domestiques* would come back to the car for more, or also rely on the feeding point, where a swannie hands out the bulging musettes. The bar closed just before the end of the stage for safety reasons – as I've said cars and bikes don't mix in red mist.

It was always a bit of a flashpoint at the feeding station. As we've said, it literally involved a swannie stretching out an arm, holding out bags for the riders to take. The problem there was forty-four outstretched arms, each team with two staff, along 200 meters of road.

Having finished the stage, it's a key time to replenish, mainly protein, which is so important in muscle recovery, because those muscles are damaged and they need protein to help in the repair process. There are various hormones that are elevated after exercise and one of them is insulin. When insulin is high, it's easier to use the protein in your diet for muscle repair, so that's why it's so important in that first hour post exercise to eat.

They may not want to. They may have an overwhelming desire to push chocolate cake into their mouth and have sugary drinks, but they'd automatically start supping the protein shake, have a meal of tuna fish or another similar protein, mixed in with some rice (or potato) for carbohydrate replenishment. It was very popular to have agave mixed with tuna, so it would be rice, tuna fish and agave in a large cinema-popcorn-sized container as the bus started to roll on to the next hotel.

So a quick snack, and they'd soon be asleep, and the music would stop the gear changes and drumming tyres of the Death Star becoming the sound track to whichever hotel we were going. Nobody cared. They just wanted a massage, food and bed. Apart from the driver, Chris Slark (Slarky), an ex-Formula One truck driver. He drove fast but carefully, never waking his passengers, never getting lost or stuck under bridges – which wasn't always the case for other teams – as the Tour crisscrossed through rural France.

Meanwhile, for the staff it was always something of a tricky situation. Mostly we acted like Napoleon, who ate the food his soldiers ate so he'd know how far he could march them; we did it out of respect and so there would be no temptations for the riders on our table. The staff would occasionally break, hopefully when the riders had left and gone to bed, and have their desserts of ice cream and cake.

24

All Shapes and Sizes

Investigating the issues around body fat with reference to riders

ATHLETES COME IN ALL SHAPES AND SIZES. Lionel Messi, perhaps the greatest footballer of all time, is five foot seven inches tall. Peter Sagan, the sprinter, is six foot, the Manx missile Mark Cavendish is five foot five inches tall, Chris Hoy six foot, Victoria Pendleton almost five foot six.

But what they all have in common is low body-fat percentage.

Weight is a performance issue in cycling, and it's obviously not just about fat. As a doctor to elite athletes I was interested in proportions, maintaining the density of bones and increasing lean muscle mass, but decreasing fat deposition.

There are two types of body fat: brown fat helps temperature regulation in newborns, while the one known to us all, white fat, is the energy store.

As I hope I've made clear, losing too much fat causes a number of other health issues as it too has other very important functions for health. It produces a hormone, leptin, which is important for metabolic rate, and produces killer T cells, part of the immune system, to fight infection.

At the other end of the scale of super skinny, is obesity. This is defined as having a BMI greater than 30 kg/m2, and after smoking it is the biggest cause of avoidable cancer deaths. It's a major risk factor in diabetes and heart disease. Team Sky and British Cycling have both made a huge contribution to the British falling in love with their bikes, increasing participation as a pastime and for commuting. Anyone who has tried to cross the cycle path along the Thames in rush hour will appreciate this. Activity can make a massive contribution to reducing obesity levels, improving the health of the nation. More and more people are getting the message: get on your bike and ride. (Or run. Or walk.)

It's mainly doctors in general practice who use BMI as a measurement to advise their patients. The body mass index was proposed by a Belgian mathematician in 1832 and is calculated by dividing the weight in kilograms by the square of the height in metres. So it doesn't measure fat exactly. In sport the gold standard is DEXA scanning – Dual-energy X-ray Absorptiometry – an X-ray body scan that lets the doctor literally see where the fat tissue is in the body – not just under the skin but around organs, and from that calculate the true percentage of body weight due to fat, muscle and bone. Fat is subcutaneous, i.e. under the skin, but also exists around the body's organs. And its this intra-abdominal (visceral) fat which is particularly harmful to health. Waist measurements have been used to assess this deposition; it's suggested that greater than 94cm in men and 80cm in women is unhealthy, greater than 102cm in men and 88cm in women is harmful.

However, at British Cycling and Team Sky we used the sum of eight skinfold measurements. This involved using skinfold calipers to take a skinfold reading, say, on the skin overlying the biceps. We'd pinch the fold of skin between the calipers and take a thickness reading in millimetres: the higher the reading the more subcutaneous fat. Add up all eight readings and that would give you a total of what we call skinfold thickness. Most would be between 40-60mm, some endurance riders would be around 35mm.

The sum of skinfolds was measured on a weekly basis, while the riders' weight was measured at least weekly in training or on a twice-daily basis (immediately after a race it especially was useful in estimating weight lost through losing fluid by sweating). We'd crunch the numbers into their spreadsheets, observing the longitudinal trends. Some riders were always on their targets for body fat, whatever the period in the season. However, others went too low and as I've said that's not a good idea. I recall taking a rider for an abdominal ultrasound scan, as I thought she had developed a hernia from weightlifting. The radiologist was typically thorough and examined not just the potential hernia sites but her organs inside; he was mesmerised by the absence of fat enveloping the organs and abdominal muscles; not his usual patient. Truly beautiful images, and I had to cough to draw him back to the task in hand.

Disciplined riders, the majority in my experience, are committed to safe and steady long-term weight-management programmes.

Reaching their optimal lean muscle mass, which is power, and the optimal amount of body fat, which is weight. It's like form, the riders feel their way there, sometimes making errors in their calculation with their coaches, but they do know eventually what the best balance is for them.

You can imagine how easy it was for riders to become weight obsessed. Anorexia was a particular worry in the academy, and there were some riders who were withdrawn from the programme in order to protect their long-term health from the serious consequences of this condition.

So what is the optimal body fat?

That's very difficult to say; but the bottom line is that if you're an elite athlete you want as little body fat as you can without running into problems.

At the same time, we – and when I say 'we' I'm really talking about the coaches – had to be careful of not pushing the athletes too hard too quickly. Coaches are performance driven, and they're success driven, and I'd often hear that awful expression from the riders, 'I'm being treated like a lump of meat!'

I don't like it when I hear that, whatever the context. These are humans with the same rights as any other patient, but of course it's a performance-driven sport, so it's fair to say that they will often be out of their comfort zone.

My role was to make sure that their programmes were safe, sustainable and not really having any long-term complications on their health. That's what the job of doctor in sports medicine is.

I started to look out for riders who were suffering in this

respect. I found that when handling a rider during examination or simply by observing them I could estimate the subcutaneous fat thickness. I could see when they were losing too much body fat. The definition of muscle groups become apparent and the veins begin to appear. In a Grand Tour, the riders are losing the battle to supply the body with enough calories to fuel the muscles, needed to power the three weeks of racing and the body starts looking for calories not just from the almost exhausted fat store but the muscles themselves. Yes, the body is eating its own muscle mass. Their appearance will look even more dramatic as the race nears the end of the third week. The riders actually do look cachexic – that's the medical term for the inevitable weight loss associated with cancer: the sunken eyes, the prominent cheek bones, the teeth that seem too big and the lollipop-sized head (the head is effectively a bony ball that doesn't shrink, but the overall body does, hence it appears to be bigger).

This brings me on to a very important subject related to weight issues, the female athlete triad. This term entered the medical literature in 1992. Occurrence of three symptoms were noted in female endurance athletes:

1. Disordered eating patterns
2. Amenorrhoea (absence of periods)
3. Increased risk of stress fractures (abnormal bone metabolism leading eventually to osteoporosis)

Calorie restriction, often to lose weight in an attempt to maximise athletic performance, results in an energy deficit, which has profound effects on the body, far wider than first thought.

This, as often happens in medicine, has led to a new descriptive term of 'relative energy deficiency in sport'. This has analogies with many health issues in elite sport, for example the relative iron deficiency issue that we touched on previously.

This deficiency has huge consequences on metabolism, menstruation and the immune system. It presents huge challenges to treat if the athlete wishes to continue elite levels of training. Rest and returning to a healthy weight by eating enough reverses the symptoms but of course this just isn't an option for the elite female athlete.

I found the adolescent academy rider new to the endurance cycling programme to be particularly at risk. The eating disorder, often subtle at first, can develop into anorexia nervosa (literally extreme weight loss by self starvation and abnormal body image) or anorexia bulimia (often maintaining weight but having an abnormal body image with binge eating and purging either by self-induced vomiting or laxatives).

These conditions are serious, life-threatening and lead to suspension or the removal of athletes from the British Cycling programme.

Such is the gravity of this situation the English Institute of Sport have developed a fast-track referral pathway to the medical experts required for treatment. As in so many other aspects of medicine, prevention is better than cure and this started with coach education and careful monitoring of weight, skin folds (the sum of eight for subcutaneous fat distribution) and close supervision by the nutritionist.

Coaches telling young riders they need to 'lose timber' trackside isn't helpful, wearing a Lycra skin suit sitting on a saddle leaves these impressionable young athletes with nowhere to hide. So my role was to protect them not just from their coaches but themselves. There are the short-term, health issues I've described, but also the longer-term ones, especially osteoporosis.

Osteoporosis is literally a thinning of the skeleton. Peak bone mass is usually 95 per cent by the age of eighteen, 99 per cent by age twenty-six provided the woman has regular periods and oestrogen production. In this syndrome the periods stop, that's called amenorrhoea, and the result is that the calcium stores needed to produce strong bones are not available. The result is a susceptibility to stress fractures, particularly of the tibia in endurance runners. The level of the calcium store thereafter slowly declines until the menopause, when loss of calcium increases. Critically these young amenorrhoeic women will start the menopause with vastly depleted levels. Optimising calcium intake and Vitamin D has not been consistently shown to improve the bone density in this group, nor has any specific drug treatment. The long-term health issue is that they develop much worse osteoporosis when they reach the menopause, with a vastly increased incidence of low impact (fragility) fractures of the hip and compression fractures in the thoracic spine (dowagers hump). As always, prevention is better than cure and I urge all young female endurance riders to eat enough calories to maintain a menstrual cycle.

Men, you don't know you're born.

25

What's Going on Upstairs?

Mental health issues in athletes

JUST LIKE ANYBODY ELSE, athletes get depressed. Certainly, I've had athletes competing on antidepressants, and I've had to withdraw riders from the intensity of their training programmes because of their mental health. Certainly, the psychological stresses professional athletes find themselves under, by their own actions and those of the team, can contribute to a mental health illness, but I think they are just humans, and anyone can suffer from depression.

As I have already discussed, I myself have suffered depression. I'd like to highlight that anyone can suffer from this, and we all have a duty to look for the symptoms and signs in our colleagues and not just shrug it off as work-related stress.

For me mental stress and ill health is another of those issues that needs debating in the open. I'm encouraged that it is now being discussed more freely in society, the Royal Princes are leading the way, and sport finally is admitting that athletes also have these health issues. The remit of even the sports medicine doctor remains holistic, and it's never just musculoskeletal problems and cardio respiratory issues that we've discussed, but also mental injury.

Because the fact is, it exists in many forms. Obviously, I'd treated many patients with a great variety of mental health issues in general practice; I never thought I'd need that skill set in professional sport. Athletes always got injured but always appeared robust. Rehabilitation is a vulnerable period, and is just as much about staying mentally well as it is getting back to play. Athletes, as I've said, often train or compete when ill or injured. Mental illness isn't as visible as a bandage, and organisations don't always want to see it, especially if the athlete is talented and still winning. I have been astounded that depression, eating disorders and self-harm don't stop success. For me, and for my patients it's never a case of winning at all costs.

Is that healthy? Does it have long-term consequences? Performance sport is a cauldron, no doubt, and you need to be able to stand the heat to play in the kitchen. Gold medals aren't given away.

There are plenty of issues around athlete welfare and protection that need to be discussed. I like to think that during my time with British Cycling I acted as a conduit – or barrier, or go-between, depending on the situation – between the athletes, the coaching staff and managers; I like to feel that I was an advocate for the athletes' long-term health, even when that went against what some coaches would have described as the immediate interests of the team. This working relationship, risk-managing the health of an athlete, is at the heart of the performance medicine and coaching model that I practised at Bolton and introduced at the velodrome. The rider allows the coach complete access to the doctor–patient consultation and is involved in health decision-making with fully informed patient consent. But I'm just one doctor, and the riders there are no longer in my care, and the fact of the matter is that this conversation still needs to take place across the sport.

26

Core Blimey

Looking at the importance of the core in cycling

WHETHER YOU'RE AN AMATEUR OR A PROFESSIONAL, you'll be aware of the importance of 'the core' in sport. It really means 'functional trunk strength', which is a better descriptive term, and when you think about it, it's common sense that the platform that the arms and legs work off in the so-called kinetic chain is strong, robust, co-ordinated and has endurance.

The 'Cinderella muscles' of sport, the back, abdomen and pelvic floor, all need conditioning, which is something that occurs during most sporting activity but specifically through targeted training, just as you'd strengthen your glutes for sprinting; it's usually done in the gym resulting in overload and adaption and better performance.

The synergistic effect of these functional trunk strength muscles is almost impossible to test, and it's impossible to have peak performance when it's missing. There's no doubt that whatever sport you're in, core stability is so important for athletic performance, and most athletes have inherent core stability. I think it's one of those things that natural-born athletes have – something denied to the likes of you and me.

It's very difficult to measure. You know when it's not there because everything seems to fall apart, since one thing's connected with another; there's a connected movement chain, the kinetic chain, and it all starts at the centre and then connects to the arms and legs.

A little time put aside two or three times a week to train the core is an essential routine for any athlete, amateur or professional. Squats, split squats, press-ups, planks, side planks, sit-up crunches and windscreen wiper exercises (have a look on YouTube) are also basics and easy to do. Combine with some muscle and soft-tissue stretching and foam-rolling after exercise.

Stretching and rolling maintain flexibility, allowing the muscles, joints and fascia to move through their range of motion needed for performance and prevents damage to the muscles, tendons, and fascia. Fascia, hardly ever mentioned but it's everywhere in the body, is the connective tissue enveloping every muscle, tendon, bone, vessel and organ. It's like cling film supporting and holding us together, and assisting gliding motion. Its function is still poorly understood but it needs a workout too for optimum musculoskeletal health, maybe even mental health. Soft-tissue massage is the best way to work on the fascia, but it's not available to all. This connective tissue massage or release is otherwise known as myofascial release.

Specific areas can be self-treated by hard balls or even tennis balls and foam roller pressure; it's a technique easy to learn, and incorporate into a stretching routine. Again, it's worth some moments of your time online in order to look up some techniques.

Each sport has its specific needs. Cyclists need to stretch the hip flexors (Bulgarian squat), the hamstrings and the gluteal muscles (Indian knot), release the iliopsoas, quads and iliotibial band.

You can also build core and perform myofascial release with yoga and Pilates. Both were introduced at Bolton and to my surprise accepted and performed without too much stick from the footballers.

Core training is marvellous for a healthy back. There's no doubt about it, back pain is a huge problem in society and also for the cyclist who spends a long time holding a stretched forward position. The back depends on its well-being by the quality of the muscles supporting it, their strength and endurance.

I always try to explain the spine as being like building blocks, the vertebrae one on top of the other, 7 in the neck, 12 in the chest, 5 in the lumbar low back sitting on the base the sacrum which forms part of the pelvis. Imagine then inflating a cuff around all these vertebrae; these muscles give the spine stability, strength and stop it toppling over. They take the load off the intervertebral shock absorbers, the discs and the motion-guiding facet joints at the posterior aspect. So the cuff, the spinal muscles, have to be trained; they have to be conditioned to become fatigue-resistant and to work in coordination.

And if you can build some strength and conditioning for spinal muscles into your training, you're in a better position to protect your back, the discs and facet joints – not just when you're exercising but sitting at your desk for eight hours.

There's a new back campaign running at the moment that is music to my ears. It informs back-pain sufferers that they need to keep moving; they need to condition and strengthen their back muscles despite the pain. Also aerobic exercise stimulates the heart to pump more blood faster around the body, sending blood to the back, not just the vital organs such as the brain, heart and liver. These important organs get the blood first, the back is far down the pecking order. Blood carries all the body's needs for healing damaged tissue, and with in-activity the back gets ignored.

So, if you're suffering from a back problem, don't shut down. Don't head for the sanctuary of your sofa and think you've got a glass back. That's the surest way to get a chronic back problem, and chronic back pain is different to acute back pain, and much harder to alleviate, which is why there's so much chronic disability from chronic back pain around. Once again prevention is better than cure.

So your back's gone. It's in spasm and it hurts low down. What do you do? You need to try and maintain that lovely curve in the lower lumbar spine whether you're lying flat, moving around, or sitting. Use a rolled-up towel to maintain this position while sitting. The position shown in the photograph is the psoas position, which produces the least stress to the lumbar discs. So rest it. Then move about to work it and increase the blood supply.

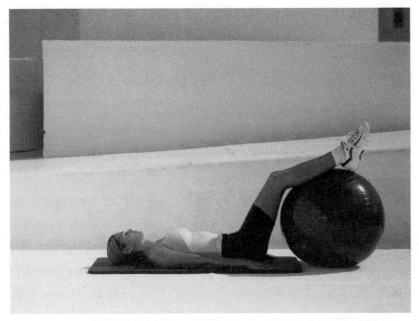

The psoas position maintaining lumbar lordosis. Compared with the pressure load on the lumbar disc in standing position this position reduces it by 50%. Bending forward and rotating increases it by 400%.

I've got nothing against even moderately strong painkillers for managing musculoskeletal pain. In hospital we used to give intravenous paracetamol to kids with fractured bones which is a very effective painkiller with very few side effects. In tablet form perhaps it's under-rated because it's over the counter, but regular paracetamol every four to six hours is very effective to allow you sufficient pain relief, to adopt the healthy postures described above but still to be able to monitor it, so you're not overdoing it by moving around too much.

Sometimes it's not enough, and the patient moves up the analgesic ladder. With increasing potency comes increasing risk of side effects. Codeine can cause constipation and affect pyscho-motor coordination. Morphine adds respiratory depression. All are addictive and dependence and misuse are prevalent issues, and not just in sport.

I try to stay on regular paracetamol, using heat and massage to settle the muscles in spasm.

An important take-home message is to try to avoid in an acute phase of injury, certainly within the first three days, non-steroidal anti-inflammatory medication. Whether you're an athlete or weekend warrior. Do not go and buy over the counter non-steroidal anti-inflammatories – ibuprofen, Nurofen – for the first three days when you snag your back or turn your ankle playing golf or football. They block the cascade of inflammation, the fundamental process by which the body heals itself.

What it does as a side-effect of blocking that cascade of inflammation is it blocks the production of the pain-generating chemicals so it feels less painful. So, great, you feel much better, but that's at the expense of the body's normal, natural healing.

Medicine is clever but the body will always be more clever. The body's always trying to heal itself and what we have to do is facilitate that, not get in the way of it.

27

A Day in the Life (part three)

It's the end of the race for our riders,
but the doctor's never off-call

THE RACE ENDS WITH A SPRINT FINISH, a dangerous time as
each team attempts to hold the road. Sometimes their sprinter
will jump on to another team's wheel. There are roundabouts,
sharp turns, street furniture, flag-waving spectators and even the
odd policeman with a camera as they race into the centre of town.

The noise increases as the barriers and hoarding get a hammering
from the screaming fans. At this point, it's best for the GC
contenders to stay out of danger.

From an organisational point of view, the finish is proper
carnage. All vehicles are diverted off the main straight some two
hundred metres from the line, and we decamp quickly in order
to get to our riders at the finish.

Poor guys. This is where you really feel for them. They've been on their bikes concentrating and racing for six hours or more, some have emptied the tank, crossed the line, only to be delivered into a whirlwind of activity: searching for teammates, their swannies with drinks. Chaperones shouting to be heard above the noise. First, second, third and a random, or targeted rider will be assigned a chaperone who will then not let them out of their sight. The rider confirms that he's been notified then has an hour to get to doping control.

Meanwhile the race organisers grab the winners, shepherding them through the crowds of journalists and cameras for the podium presentation; the TV schedule won't wait, and there's time pressure on the riders to clean up and put on clean kit, helped by their ever loyal swannie, which of course they have to do in the presence of a chaperone, because of the doping control.

Next the winner's whisked off to do press, *blah, blah, blah*, I'm silently saying to them, 'Come on, come on, we need to get a move on.'

Doping control needs 90ml of urine, which is hard if the rider's dehydrated. Gulping down 2 litres isn't the answer as then there's a rush of dilute urine – too diluted and it's rejected. Then there's going to be a long wait.

It's an ideal time for a protein shake. The 'golden hour' has begun – the hour during which they should be replenishing stores of protein and carbohydrate.

Often there's only one anti-doping officer, which can hold the whole process up. And when you've got to go you've got to go.

A Day in the Life (part three)

The riders have mutual respect, it's not always done first in first out. It is also a haven from the press and time for quiet banter.

At the same time, others are trying to catch up with them, the team's press officer, independent journalists. Will they talk further to the press?

It's noisy, it's busy, there are people rushing around everywhere, and you're at the Tour de France, no other bike race comes close to it – but still, we're thinking ahead, we're thinking of getting the athletes treated, and fed and then tucked up in bed ready for tomorrow's stage.

And it's vitally important that we do it. In the past, Brailsford has been known to hire a helicopter to get the GC off a mountain-top finish fast.

If the next hotel is down in the valley the riders jump on their bikes simply because it's quicker than using the bus. Usually it's an hour's drive away. The driver has already planned the route, the satnav is programmed, and he knows how long it's going to take, so we can phone ahead to tell our people when to expect us. Most of the staff are already there at the hotel, never seeing the finish. Those who have nothing to do with the race moved on at first light to prepare. The mechanic's truck goes ahead to get a prime spot in the car park. That is first come first served, and competitive. *Soigneurs* hoover the rooms, set up the beds, all that sleep hygiene stuff, and the chef will have gone to look at the kitchens.

And now we're trying to get the riders on to the bus, 'Come on, come on,' and it's with their best interests in mind because they don't want to be rude to the public or press (well, in most cases) but they've got us hassling them, and most of all they're absolutely bloody knackered.

They climb on to the bus. If it's been a good day, the atmosphere's great, lots of banter, very euphoric. If it's been a bad day they're like dead men walking. That's the difference in psychology. When you're winning you have so much more energy and resilience. Losing batters you mentally. You've put all that physical effort in, to little reward.

The ones who finish first jump in the shower first. There are two shower heads in the cubicle so they go in two at a time, a queue forming behind them. All use the Betadine antiseptic surgical scrubbing brush to clean their road rash. These professionals usually do a good job, but if I see them struggling I'll do it for them and accept their cursing. Quite simply that first clean is the most important for rapid healing. Out comes grit and dirt. Out they come, towelling themselves off and heading to the back of the bus where we have two opposing benches. Here they jump on the scales so I can get a post-race weight. Road rash dressings, saddle sores too. At the same time I'm assessing them for the later treatment needs at the next hotel.

If we're lucky they won't need anything too drastic, but it's hardly unknown: Geraint Thomas rode the 2013 Tour de France with a fractured pelvis. Others have lacerations to suture, have suffered fractured vertebrae, fractured ribs, or concussive symptoms and these obviously need initial diagnosis, later a management plan with my travelling support team, informed consent to the risks of continuing and so forth. It might be that we have to take them off for an imaging procedure, usually an MR scan at a local hospital, which offers something of a challenge. The race organisers are really good when it comes to dealing with acute trauma needing abandonment, and will help with X-rays and trips to A&E. However, obtaining an MR scan is more difficult. Team jerseys are a vital currency in opening up scanning departments.

Hopefully we won't need hospital visits. Mainly I'm dealing with overuse injuries. That's why physiotherapists and the soft-tissue therapists are such an important part of the team. The riders' musculoskeletal systems have taken a pounding and they need at least an hour of soft-tissue treatment with their swannie and then with the physiotherapist back at the hotel.

Patched up, they go back to their seats, where after four or five hours riding with their legs 'dependent', in other words below the heart, their legs will be swollen with tissue fluid and feel uncomfortable.

The seats on the Death Star are specially designed for the athletes, in order that they can lie almost flat and especially to elevate their legs. It helps with aching and fluid return.

All riders will pull on their compression tights, a must for all serious amateur athletes, as discussed. More serious musculoskeletal injuries are immediately treated with the ice compression cuffs around the affected part to limit the swelling.

Prevention of swelling, which is necessary for recovery of function (hence the RICE first aid treatment we all know) is much easier than trying to deal with it later. Instant ice packs and strapping of difficult-to-cuff anatomical parts conclude the on-bus care. The bus keeps on rolling, and I move to the front jockey seat attempting to control my motion sickness.

There's a small kitchen on the bus and we make sure the riders, having taken protein shakes, continue refuelling with real food, protein and carbs within that golden hour, and of course continue to rehydrate.

If we are lucky, it's a transfer of an hour, if we're unlucky, it's three hours, moving ever closer to Paris.

Arriving at the hotel, our forward party is waiting for us, probably having got up the noses of the hotel staff. A swannie hands out room key cards and gives riders the all-important wi-fi passcode. A little touch, a little marginal gain, no trooping down to reception. They're told exactly where to go to find their rooms, where the swannies' bedrooms (massage) rooms are, which one is the food room and of course where the doc's room is, and where dinner will be served.

We always make sure that riders, swannies and doc are roomed close together so there can be some cross-contact but also so they're close to the food room, which is actually a *soigneur*'s bedroom, left open so that riders can wander in and graze on nuts, dried fruit, cereal, and a scoop of protein powder.

Nearby also? Me. So if they need me they know immediately where to find me, and I know where they are for the morning doping control. Like the food room, I also operate an open-door policy. Literally, the door is ajar so that riders can walk in, and chat and it's only closed for consultation and treatment.

They unwind with music or watching road cycling on TV, or chatting on the phone; at the same time the *soigneur* attempts to work wonders on their muscles and soft tissues. The riders form a close bond with their *soigneur*.

A Day in the Life (part three)

Now it's time for the evening meal, where the riders all sit down together for a starter of salad and olive oil, a vegetable smoothie followed by chicken, salmon and rice, maybe potatoes with as many green vegetables as they like, very little pasta or bread and fruit for dessert and then coffee. And they eat a lot – needing those 5,000-6,000 calories a day.

There's no alcohol, of course. No rider would drink alcohol during a Grand Tour, but as for the staff, at Team Sky we operated a different policy to the one that was in force at British Cycling. At Team Sky there's a more continental feel; as it's part of eating there is occasionally some red wine on offer, although if it has been a stage win or jersey there will be champagne.

Funnily enough, one of the things that struck me about my time in British Cycling was that we didn't really know how to celebrate properly.

Football, rugby, Formula One – teams will party for days after significant victories, but that was never the case either in British Cycling or Team Sky. There was the odd sip of champagne, but that was about it. And please don't think that I regret that because I'm an inveterate party animal, not at all, but it was a missed opportunity for team-building and morale.

Riders are incredibly disciplined athletes. Like any professional athlete, they have to make sacrifices and one of those is alcohol. Why? Because it's empty calories. It's not protein, it's not fat, it's carbohydrate and leads simply to fat stores and weight gain. When a rider's finding it difficult to maintain weight, it's usually not from pizza but because they're drinking too much alcohol in my experience and that needs to be sensitively addressed and talked over.

Mainly, though, they simply don't. And even when they toast a rider, they usually take a sip and then leave it, they wouldn't finish the glass.

After the meal, Yates, the *directeur sportif*, swings round to the rider's rooms to ask how they're feeling and to discuss race tactics and ask for tomorrow's gears. Mostly he'll find them lying on their beds with their feet up the wall, in the 'reverse dependent' posture. Later, they can expect a visit from me as I do my 'ward round', making any final dressing checks and gently advising them to get off their phones and laptop screens.

And that's it. Lights out. Ready to do it all again the next day.

28

Triumph, Acclaim

How to deal with winning
(but mostly how to deal with losing)

IT COULD OFTEN BE DAYS AFTER A MAJOR RACE when defeat would hit a rider.

It's very difficult to know how to deal with somebody when they haven't succeeded; when they've been training so, so hard, they've given it their all, they've found form, and yet still been beaten by their rivals, often a particular nemesis, particularly in the limited pool of track riders. Of course it's not always accurate to say that if you don't succeed you fail, because there's a whole lot of ground in between, but even so, that's how many riders think of it, especially those in the track squad, where it's usually head-to-head.

It's a bit different for the road riders, of course. Their purpose is to race as a team, and it's up to the *domestiques* to support the

GC. Crashes often end a challenge in the Tour and whilst not all can be prevented it's the road captain's role to marshal the *domestiques* to ride around the GC, protecting his hard-fought space in the peloton.

It's an approach that can sometimes backfire. There was a flashpoint during stage 11 of the 2012 Tour de France, where Froome was leading Wiggins up to the mountain finish at the now infamous La Toussuire. Wiggins was suffering. Froome was on it and burst ahead but obviously on his race radio came something along the lines of 'help Brad' as Sean Yates, the *directeur sportif* explained in his autobiography (I wasn't there).

That incident was probably the start of the split between Wiggins and Froome.

Could Chris Froome have won the 2012 Tour de France? I think it's highly probable. However, Bradley Wiggins was the chosen one, he was the GC and those were the team orders. Froome was professional to agree.

Next year Froome was given the chance to ride as GC in the 2013 Tour and the rest is history. It's the team principal who decides the GC, not the riders.

During most of my time at Sky the team was built around Wiggins. When he left, it was built around Froome. Cavendish left too; his dream was to be a sprinter with another green jersey and he knew he had to move to a less GC-dominant team. It was a pity as the British icons began to melt away.

Sure cycling is a team sport but it doesn't always seem like that with the podium for three. They are hard men who empty the tank and yet they remain out of the spotlight. They certainly earned my respect on the Grand Tours, especially the immense engine that is the unassuming Ian Stannard, who won Omloop Het Nieuwsblad two years running.

Geraint Thomas, another hard man, is more than capable of a GC win and I hope he soon gets the opportunity.

But as for those riders who come home without the hoped-for jerseys or medals, there were a lot of staff who didn't know how to deal with it. I'd see a situation where riders and coaching staff would fall silent, unable to look me or anybody else in the eye. They'd be looking at the floor, absolutely gutted. Devastated.

It was Dr Peters, actually, who gave me advice on how to deal with defeat. 'Richard, *you* can't ignore it,' he said, 'because everybody else will.'

I knew what he meant. A rider would often seem to wear a shroud of defeat. It would affect the way that other people interacted with them, as though their lack of success might somehow be catching. You'd have a situation where the coaches couldn't even talk to them, let alone other members of staff, such as *soigneurs* and mechanics.

What I learned from Dr Peters was *not* to be one of those people. Go to the rider, put a hand on their shoulder, try and establish eye contact if you can, and say, 'Is there anything I can do? Do you need anything?'

Usually that would be the beginning of a very quiet conversation about something and nothing: 'Yeah, I could do with a towel' or, 'I could do with a drink, Doc,' after which it was a just a case of getting things moving, get the rider changed, get them to begin recovery if it was a stage race, which was important if they'd lost a lot of time, because then they needed to get going, rest, recover and prepare for the next day.

The same in the Olympic Games, a rider would sometimes have another event, so they had to start getting their head together.

Dr Peters always advised me that there were those who were looking for someone to blame. However, his advice was, *That's okay*. Try and make it so that they don't blame themselves. They should blame outside influences. Otherwise they're looking deep into their own psyche and they end up feeling that they have got a fault or a weakness. Thus it's much better to think, 'The other team were better than me,' than, 'I was worse than them,' or to blame the bike, the wheels, the track, the temperature, the heat, the man with the dog at the side of the road. Looking for a future gain.

Sure enough, that was my general approach. But at the same time it was also very individual. Some people would shrug it off and be happy-go-lucky, the joker. Others would be so introspective and just beat themselves up.

For example, Victoria Pendleton always took her battles with Anna Meares very seriously. But Dr Peters was her talisman. It just goes to show how important he was.

When the riders bought into his mind-management programme, they really bought into it and this ensured another personal marginal gain. This programme is eloquently described in his book, *The Chimp Paradox*. Indeed his input pre-race was so crucial that in the run up to London 2012, Dr Peters was *the* essential member of the travelling support staff. Sir Chris Hoy stated that 'the mind programme helped me win my gold medals'. Victoria Pendleton went further, saying, 'Steve Peters is the most important person in my career.'

After winning gold at London 2012 it was Dr Peters she collapsed on, crying her heart out. That was to be her final race and the years of tension and stress just flowed out.

You could always tell when Wiggins was on top of it and relaxed or winning, because he would do impersonations of you. But on the other hand, if he hadn't succeeded, then he was best left well alone.

He would go through the motions of recovery but he didn't need to talk about it and he often roomed on his own, because the Tour de France team was nine riders, which boiled down to four lots of two, plus Bradley on his own.

So he'd retreat into his room and have his massage, he'd probably come down to eat early or late, to miss his teammates and then when I did my last ward round at night when I was going round checking everyone was okay, I'd knock on his door and often there wouldn't be an answer.

In the early days, I was concerned, I used to knock and think, *Oh no, is he in trouble?* I'd text him and there'd be no answer.

I remember his last race for Team Sky. It didn't go the way he wanted, and there was no real post-race celebration of all his achievements at Team Sky, nor any proper send-off from Brailsford, which upset him. In fact, he ended up spending the night in a different hotel from the rest of us as no one had told him anything was being put on for him.

*   *   *

The Line

It was always particularly difficult when somebody had lost through injury. Because the feeling of loss is a psychological feeling, when you put that together with physical pain, either extensive road rash or even a fractured clavicle or worse, that was like a double whammy and it was difficult. And there was the road to rehabilitation to face.

At the football club, when the team had played badly and lost, sometimes the manager didn't even come down to the changing room and instead of travelling back on the coach, or going to the airport, travelling back with us, he'd travel back alone with his own thoughts.

Sometimes when we'd lost they'd take it to the dressing room, incredibly subdued, or there would be a flare-up about whose turn it was in the showers, little fire fights would start, retribution and blame.

People are a lot more prepared to deal with success and talking to the media, sharing it, celebrating, so there's a lot of ways of dealing with success but not many ways of dealing with failure. In cycling, as I've already said, we didn't really 'do' celebration that well; there was none at British Cycling and at Team Sky there would be a rapping of a spoon on a glass and everyone would stand up with a glass of champagne and make a sound, a very traditional noise in cycling, a crescendo of 'Whooooo,' and then sit down.

Funny thing was, most of the people in the room didn't even drink.

29

The Finishing Line

Looking back, what do I take from my time in cycling?

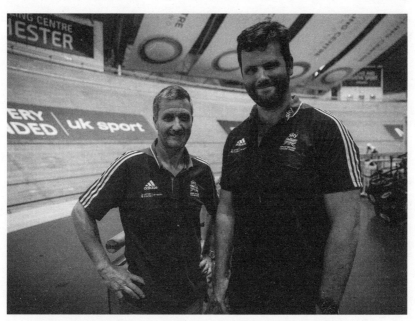

Myself with Phil Burt, an exceptionally talented physiotherapist and
bike fit expert, now ex-British Cycling.

WHEN I WAS FIRST OFFERED A JOB in cycling I told a colleague about my career move.

He looked at me askance.

'Are you mad?' he said, 'think of your professional reputation.'

I was reminded of those words during 2017, when I found myself the focus of unwelcome media attention. A journalist 'doorstepped' me – though thankfully not on my actual doorstep – and I was suddenly a fixture of the newspapers. 'Today's papers are tomorrow's chip wrapping,' was what they used to say. But that's no longer true in this digital age. Today's news is tomorrow's Google search term. For all the reasons that we've discussed – and I've been as honest as I know how – I felt that my name had been dragged through the mud. As Dwight D. Eisenhower once said, 'The search for the scapegoat is the easiest of hunting expeditions.'

Nevertheless, even though I can't deny a slightly bitter taste in my mouth, I can look back at my time with British Cycling and Team Sky fondly, confident in the knowledge that although I didn't do everything right – my record-keeping, my failure to back up my data – I did a lot that *was* right.

And I know that I did it clean, and without ever crossing the line.

I know, also, that I helped shape a genuinely new and innovative approach to sports science, 'Performance Health Management', where we combined the performance demands of the team with the health management of the riders, balancing short- and long-term risk factors, practising informed consent and preaching athlete preference, making informed 'return to play' decisions.

What's more it was an approach that worked. I am the first to admit – indeed it's a bugbear of mine as you've probably guessed – that professional sport can be unhealthy but I fought hard to make sure that any short-term drawbacks never became longer-term problems. I tried to see to it, that the relationship between medicine and sport remained a balanced one. True, the demands of the sport meant that occasionally I would have to rely on medicine in order to meet athlete preference. Triamcinolone is a good example. Would I use it as much in general medical practice? Probably not. Would I use it again in a performance-driven environment? Yes. Is it bad medicine? I don't think so, but that doesn't necessarily make it good medicine either. It was just the right medicine at the time.

I tried to ensure that athletes never leaned too heavily on medicine at the expense of the basics: hydration, nutrition, recovery, sleep and good hygiene.

Mainly, I know that I abided by my core principles to 'do no harm', and kept to the belief that it's not about winning at all costs, and I did that by remaining firm in my conviction that those in my care were patients before they were professional athletes, and should be extended the same rights governing any doctor–patient relationship. They have the right to receive the same treatment as an ordinary member of the public. This is why TUEs are necessary, although I think we have to constantly review the WADA code and see to it that we are always working to improve the quality of analytical testing and prevent the abuse of good medicines in the pursuit of performance in sport.

In the meantime, I hope I've given the amateur some tips, not just ideas to incorporate into their own training adaptations, but to improve their overall health. A free-to-access website linked to the book, will soon be launched. This will provide resources about the major issues, screening for sudden cardiac death, and assessing concussion, through to stretching, core exercises and road rash management. All in one easily accessible place, not for the pros, but for you, the enthusiastic amateur.

Because at the end of the day, exercise should be fun and has immense health gains. I'm proud to have been associated with the increased levels of cycling, enjoyable physical activity that the achievements of our athletes have ignited.

As a nation, we should be proud of our sporting heroes and their achievements. Personally, I'm very proud of what we at Team Sky and British Cycling achieved in terms of our nation's health gains. Go out at the weekend and you'll see hordes of cyclist on the roads. Cyclists of all ages and abilities enjoying a fun, sociable, healthy activity. Perhaps this is the true legacy of Dave Brailsford and his marginal gains, of Bradley Wiggins, Chris Froome, Chris Hoy, Victoria Pendleton and Laura Trott. Certainly I'm very proud of my part in it, and I hope it continues.

Lastly, as a doctor, I ask you just one favour. Enjoy living healthily. Enjoy your cycling. But just make sure you leave '*chute!*' out of it.

The Finishing Line

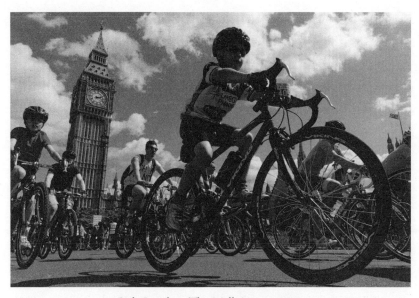

Ride London, The Mall August 2013.
I'm proud of my part in it and hope it continues.

Appendix 1

Skin Health for Female Cyclists

*The following is the text of a Powerpoint presentation given
by consultant dermatologist Dr Jane Sterling, who worked
with us on Project Ouch*

THE SKIN AND SUBCUTANEOUS TISSUES take a lot of trauma
during cycling, so keeping everything in as good shape as possible
is essential for comfort and therefore performance.

Just as you look after your muscles and joints, so you need to
look after the skin 'down there'.

Know what is normal for you
Use a mirror to have a look at your normal genital anatomy and
colour of skin.

WHY?
Because you will then know when it changes or when it does not
look right.

People who carry more fat increase the fatty tissue in the mons
pubis, labia majora and buttocks. If you do not carry much fat
on the body then these areas are less 'padded'.

If you might normally get sore, itchy or feel cracks or bumps in the skin, it would be a good idea to have your skin examined by a doctor.

WHY?

There are some skin conditions that can affect the skin of the genital area. If you do have any of these conditions and don't know about it, then the trauma of cycling will definitely make things worse. Thrush is very common and if not treated properly can cause a prolonged but mild skin irritation. Reactions to applications can also cause low-grade skin inflammation and reduced skin barrier function.

Understand how the skin works, protects itself and repairs itself

WHY?

Because then you can do the best to keep your skin in tip-top condition.

The genital skin is a micro-environment. The area tends to feels sweaty and because there is not so much open circulation of air, the skin and air around the area are often humid.

The area is naturally smelly, like armpits, as the sweat glands in these areas produce a slightly different sweat to the rest of the body.

The area is hairy – hair helps protect the sensitive skin and also helps the sweat to evaporate more quickly.

The crotch area is not a particularly greasy area, but there are grease glands (sebaceous glands) that produce a little oil to help maintain the surface and water resistance of the skin. Washing with soapy cleaners removes this and so removes the natural protective layer on the skin.

Basic skin care

Keep the skin clean but not over-clean

WHY?

All skin carries bacteria on it all the time and the ano-genital area carries a slightly different collection of skin bacteria to somewhere like the back or thighs. If you remove too many of the usual bacteria, then other less desirable bacteria will move in.

How?

If you can, clean and rinse the skin with plain water after opening the bowels. Ideally use a bidet or shower. Don't scrub. Use a soap or washing liquid if you like, once or at most twice a day, but the most important step is to rinse all detergent-type products off afterwards. You can use a perfume-free moisturiser as a washing cream instead (e.g. Dermol 500).

Keep the skin as dry as possible

WHY?

Very damp skin against fabric will often lead to increased chafing. When you exercise, you often notice the sweating when you stop moving.

How?

If you could shower soon after exercise to wash away the sweat, cool down a little and then dress in loose clothes, the skin could be less likely to chafe during the post-cycling period.

Improve the barrier function of the skin

WHY?

If the skin is dry and flaky, it has a reduced barrier function. This means that irritants (like soap, shower gel, sweat, preserving agents in creams, shampoos etc.) can penetrate the surface of the skin and set up an inflammation. This in turn makes the skin lose its barrier function and be more susceptible to the irritants and the skin is more likely to suffer chafing due to friction.

How?

Allow the skin to keep its natural layer of moisturiser – so don't wash too often. Once a day is enough. If you have to wash more than that, do not use soap or shower gel on the sensitive areas. A soft moisturiser like Dermol 500 or Neutrogena Body Lotion as a soap substitute may be used. Avoid rubbing the skin with a flannel, sponge or exfoliator. Dry by patting, use a cool hairdryer or allow to dry naturally. Apply a little moisturiser after the skin is dry.

Anyone can become allergic to the chemicals in creams, even if they have been using them for a long time. Creams contain all sorts of things: preservatives to stop them going off, plant extracts, chemicals to alter the consistency etc. You should test a new cream out by applying it to exactly the same area on the soft skin of your inner forearm daily for a week before using it on the sensitive areas. If the daily application to the forearm does not lead to a red, itchy or sore reaction, then it is probably okay to use on the genital area.

Don't shave

WHY?

Shaving causes small nicks in the skin – wet shaving is worst, but dry shaving also damages the surface of the skin.

Depilatory creams contain chemicals that dissolve the keratin in hair so that it softens and can be scraped off. The surface of the skin is the epidermis, which is also made of keratin layers, so that the creams will dissolve away the very surface skin cells too. Because normal skin does repair itself after using a depilatory cream within a couple of days, for most people this does not have a major effect, but if you are also rubbing away the surface of the skin due to friction of clothing, then the skin could become quite sore.

Pulling out hairs by waxing, threading or using an epilator can also damage the skin surface and does damage the hair root as the hair is pulled out.

Laser hair removal also damages the hair root, but perhaps more gently than by pulling the hairs out.

If you feel you have to remove pubic and groin hair, the best would be to leave a comfortably soft length of hair (longer than stubble) either by trimming carefully with scissors or by using a beard trimmer with a guard.

What can be done to prevent/minimise chafing during a long ride / tour?

2 weeks before the ride: Check skin

2–4 days before the ride: use a light moisturiser that suits you, apply morning and evening, This will help to ensure that the barrier function of the skin is in good shape.

On the day, wash gently (no rubbing or scrubbing) with moisturising wash. Dry gently (again no rubbing) – pat or use a cold hairdryer.

Use something on the skin to decrease friction of the skin – a silicon-containing application (e.g. Bodyglide, Chamois butter, Sprilon spray), a heavy greasy application (e.g. Vaseline, Epaderm etc).

Shorts, chamois insert and saddle may all contribute to chafing, so make sure they are a good fit for you.

If you have a long body and your suit pulls tight in the groin, on each side, this will make it likely to chafe in the groin crease. If you have wider thighs and there is not enough lateral stretch in the shorts, there may be increased pull of material in the groin, leading to a line of chafing.

The chamois insert needs to be the right shape to fit your width and length of undercarriage, and width of thighs. If the fit is not good, it may bend/fold in such a way that a small area of increased pressure rubs on the skin and chafes.

The saddle also needs to be a good fit for your width of undercarriage and where you tend to sit on the saddle.

After the ride, remove shorts, and wash as above as soon as possible. Wash skin gently. Apply a rich but simple moisturiser immediately after washing to increase the barrier function of the skin.

You may find that loose silky underwear is comfortable to wear (e.g. Dermasilk).

How best to recover after chafing

Prolonged friction to the skin literally rubs away the surface layers of the epidermis. As the most superficial layers go, the barrier function of the skin is impaired and the skin reacts by getting red and feeling sensitive. It will then be more prone to be irritated by sweat and chemicals. As more of the surface is rubbed away, the skin may develop oozing – this is because the natural tissue fluids can leak outwards from the impaired barrier of the skin. This is much more painful at the site of the erosion. This will ooze for a while and then dry up with a crust. If the friction continues, the skin may bleed as blood vessels near the surface break and the blood also leaks out. This will dry to a scab.

If no more friction occurs, the skin will repair itself. If the skin has broken to oozing or bleeding, it will take a week or two for the skin to look back to normal, but another 2–3 weeks for the skin strength to return. Maximise healing by eating well, sleeping, etc. Wash with plain water, apply a soothing cream – a mild antiseptic like Savlon may suit, or a plain light moisturiser. Continue to wear clothes that are loose.

Minimize bruising

Bumpy rides can cause bruising or more troublesome injury

WHY?

Bumping of the body on a hard object can cause a bruise. A bruise is caused by damaged blood vessels which then leak blood into the soft tissues causing the colour to change from purple (fresh blood) to yellow/brown as the blood is broken down and cleared away by the body's immune cells. If the bumping injury is severe the blood leakage may be a more obvious bleed into the soft tissue under the surface, a haematoma. This may need a small operation to drain the collection of blood.

Severe injury of this sort may also damage the lymph vessels. The lymph vessels or lymphatics drain tissue fluid away and eventually back into the blood stream. The lymphatics do not repair themselves easily and if they are damaged/not working properly, this can lead to chronic swelling of the damaged area, called lymphoedema.

How?

When you can, reduce contact between a hard saddle and the vulva. This might mean increasing padding to the saddle with a gel or foam saddle cover during e.g. time on the rollers, training on a static cycle.

What application to reduce friction is best?

Whatever works for you and does not produce a bad reaction on your skin. All creams and sprays, including those designed to be anti-friction, contain several constituents which could irritate skin or could produce an allergy. These potential problem constituents include solvents (e.g. propylene glycol, alcohol), preservatives (e.g. phenoxyethanol, butylated hydroxyanisole, quarternium 15, imidazolidinyl urea), agents which alter consistency (e.g. emulsifiers and stabilisers such as cetearyl alcohol, octyldodecanol), chemicals to mask the smell of other ingredients (e.g. menthol, fragrances), and plant and animal products (e.g. beeswax, lanolin).

If you can apply a cream to the same place on the sensitive skin of the inner arm every day for 7 days and it does not cause a red, itchy or sore skin reaction, then the cream is probably safe for you to use.

Appendix 2

Cardiopulmonary Resuscitation (CPR): When to Use It And What to Do

The basics

Cardiopulmonary resuscitation, or CPR, is a means of preserving life in a patient in cardiac arrest. No doubt you've seen it done on TV and in films. But where the movies get it wrong is that CPR cannot 'restart' the heart. In fact, its principal function is to send blood to the brain and heart, thus delaying tissue death and hopefully preventing brain damage. Defibrillation is needed in order to restore a heart rhythm.

When to use it

Use CPR when a patient is in cardiac arrest, in other words, when they are unconscious, not breathing and their heart is not working. If this is the case then you need to do two things: firstly, phone for an ambulance; secondly, perform what we call 'hands-on' CPR.

How to do it

Press down hard on the breast bone, and then to the beat of the song '500 Miles' by The Proclaimers – or, if you're of a more disco persuasion, to the beat of the song 'Stayin' Alive' by the Bee Gees – begin to make compressions, two per second, making 30 in all, followed by two rescue breaths. And then repeat.

What next?

Go online and look at some videos. Better still, attend a course and get trained in basic CPR. You could save a life.

Appendix 3

Recognising Concussion: A Quick Guide for Coaches and Officials

The basics

If a bang to the heads *looks* bad it probably *is bad*, and may well have caused concussion. Loss of consciousness is perhaps the biggest red flag but please bear in mind that a patient doesn't have to have been unconscious in order to have a concussion injury.

How to recognise it

In the first instance, be on the lookout for a patient who is motionless and slow to get up. In football it was always the case that we doctors worried less about a player who was writhing on the floor, seemingly in agony, than one who lay still. Clearly, if the patient is clutching their head, that's also a bad sign.

After that, any of the following indicates a possible concussion:

Convulsions / fit / twitching

Unsteady on feet / falling over / poor coordination

Confusion

Disorientation

Dazed, blank and / or vacant look

Meanwhile, be alert for worrying symptoms, such as a severe

and worsening headache, or 'pressure' in the head; visual problems, the patient feeling as though they're 'in a fog' and unable to concentrate, nausea and vomiting, and any other unusual behaviour. Please also be vigilant for associated neck injury – in other words, severe neck pain, weakness, tingling burning or a numb sensation in the arms and legs.

Try and further establish concussion injury with the following questions.
Where are we?
What time of day is it?
Who are we playing / what race is this?
Who did we play / race last and who won?
What's my name?

What to do about it
If any of these observations are present or the answers are incorrect then it's time to remove the sportsperson from the event and seek medical advice. Remember: if in doubt sit them out.

What next?
As before, go online and familiarise yourself with the signs and symptoms. Again, why not attend a course?

Appendix 4

Nigel Mitchell's Rice Cakes

As we've said throughout the book, our nutritionist Nigel Mitchell's rice cakes were the stuff of legend and an essential addition to the musettes used during the Grand Tours. Not only were they nutritious and delicious, but they helped to wash out the unpleasant taste of the various bars and gels the riders consumed. What's more it didn't melt in their jerseys. Here's the recipe . . .

Ingredients
500g Arborio rice
750ml water
300g Philadelphia cheese
400g Nutella

1. Throw the water and rice into a rice cooker and boil until the water is gone.
2. Stir in the Philadelphia and three quarters of the Nutella.
3. Pop the mix into a medium-sized zip lock bag and lay flat as a slab.
4. When cool, place it into the fridge overnight.
5. In the morning, cut the slab into bite-sized pieces.

Appendix 5

Road Rash

1. Rinse the wound as soon as possible with copious amounts of tap water.
2. Clean the wound under a warm shower as soon as practically possible. Use a soft nail brush and povidone iodine antiseptic to remove as much gravel and debris as you can. THIS IS THE MOST IMPORTANT STEP.
3. Cover with a non-adherent dressing. You'd ideally have some hydropolymer or hydrocolloid dressings in your first-aid kit. Leave undisturbed for 48 hours. These dressings absorb the large amount of tissue fluid produced during this first stage of healing – the exudative stage.
4. After 48 hours allow the wound to be exposed to the fresh air as much as possible to facilitate healing.
5. If there is increasing pain, redness, heat or swelling at the site of the wound seek medical advice.

Appendix 6

Therapeutic Use Exemption Guidelines: Hay Fever

APPLICATIONS MUST BE SUBMITTED IN ADVANCE of treatment and be supported by medical evidence to justify therapeutic use.

Required supporting evidence:

1. Description of symptoms to confirm diagnosis

Provide details of when the hay fever started; the symptoms experienced; the severity of these symptoms; the effect on performance; and symptoms suffered in previous years.

2. Medical history documented

Provide details of any known allergens or allergic history. Submit results of immunological investigations such as skin prick tests or specific IgE to confirm these details.

3. Confirmation that reasonable therapeutic alternatives have been trialled

Provide details of the permitted oral, nasal and/or ophthalmic medications that have been trialled for at least 2 weeks including names, doses, dates, duration and the effect of the treatment.

4. Specialist referral

A specialist opinion (i.e. ENT, immunologist or respiratory) is required to support the proposed treatment request. The specialist will need to give a reasoned opinion in view of the British Society for Allergy and Clinical Immunology (BSACI) guidelines and NHS Clinical Knowledge Summaries (CKS) on hay fever.

Taken from UK Anti-Doping guidelines, as were applicable 2011–2015 inclusive.

Bradley Wiggins,
Paris-Roubaix 2015

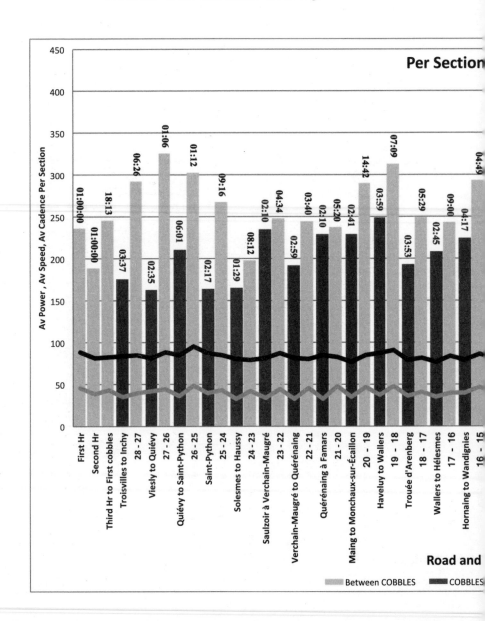

Per Section

Av Power , Av Speed, Av Cadence Per Section

Between COBBLES	COBBLES

Road and

This graph shows the speed, pedal cadence and power exerted by Bradley Wiggins during Paris-Roubaix 2015. The light grey bars indicate the sections of the race that took place on road, the dark grey is on cobbles.

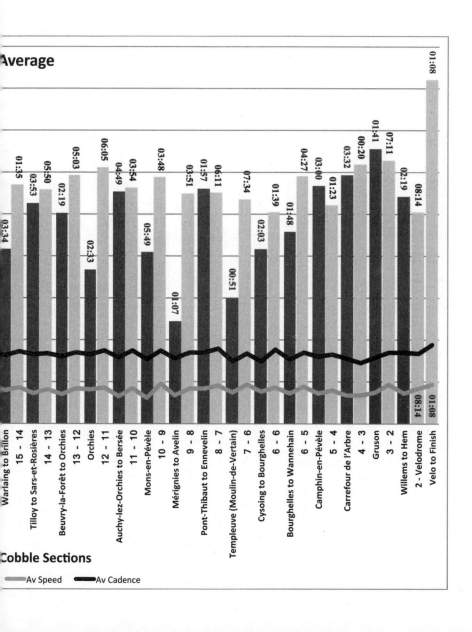

Average

Section	Value
Warlaing to Brillon	03:34
15 – 14	01:35
Tilloy to Sars-et-Rosières	03:53
14 – 13	05:50
Beuvry-la-Forêt to Orchies	02:19
13 – 12	05:03
Orchies	02:33
12 – 11	06:05
Auchy-lez-Orchies to Bersée	04:49
11 – 10	03:54
Mons-en-Pévèle	05:49
10 – 9	03:48
Mérignies to Avelin	01:07
8 – 9	03:51
Pont-Thibaut to Ennevelin	01:57
8 – 7	06:11
Templeuve (Moulin-de-Vertain)	00:51
7 – 6	07:34
Cysoing to Bourghelles	02:03
6 – 6	01:39
Bourghelles to Wannehain	01:48
6 – 5	04:27
Camphin-en-Pévèle	03:00
5 – 4	01:23
Carrefour de l'Arbre	03:32
4 – 3	00:20
Gruson	01:41
3 – 2	07:11
Willems to Hem	02:19
2 – Velodrome	08:14
Velo to Finish	01:08

Cobble Sections

▬▬Av Speed ▬▬▬Av Cadence

Photo Credits

Acknowledgements

Thanks must go to my father for telling me that evil flourishes when good men do nothing; to my father-in-law, who taught me that when the going get tough, the tough get going; to my tutors and colleagues in medicine; to my mentors in professional sport, Sam Allardyce, Mark Taylor, Sir Dave Brailsford and Dr Steve Peters; to my psychiatrist Dr Saleem; to Andrew Holmes and Alex Clarke at Wildfire Publishing; to Richard Thompson, my agent at M&C Saatchi; and finally, and most importantly, to my family.

Index

320

Index

Index